EMERSON THE BRAVE

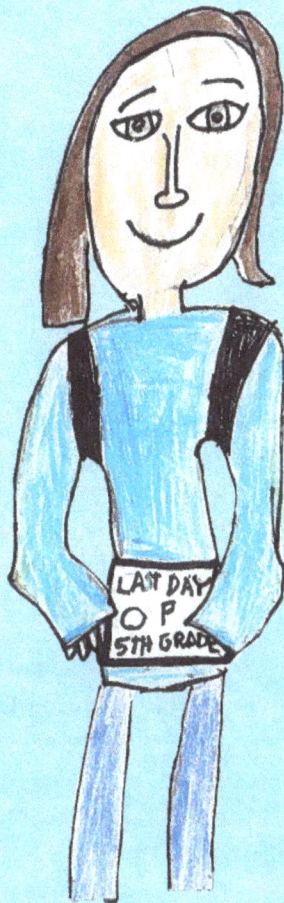

LAST DAY
O P
5TH GRADE

ILLUSTRATED BY EMERSON HOOGENDOORN, AVERY FRANCIS, CHRISTIAN BRADLEY, ELENA DE ALVARE, KORA HOISINGTON, AND URIJAH TAYLOR

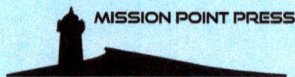

MISSION POINT PRESS

Published by Mission Point Press
2554 Chandler Rd.
Traverse City, MI 49696
(231) 421-9513
www.MissionPointPress.com

Edited by Julie Kovacs
Book design by Sarah Meiers

ISBN: 978-1-965278-06-2
Library of Congress Control Number: 2024921170

Printed in the United States of America

EMERSON
- THE -
BRAVE

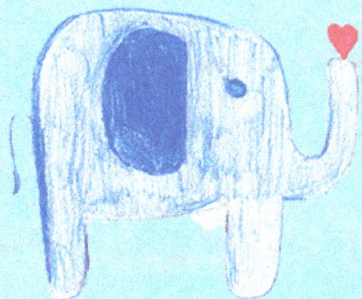

MY CANCER JOURNEY FROM A-Z

EMERSON HOOGENDOORN

ILLUSTRATED BY EMERSON HOOGENDOORN, AVERY FRANCIS, CHRISTIAN BRADLEY, ELENA DE ALVARE, KORA HOISINGTON, AND URIJAH TAYLOR

EDITED BY JULIE KOVACS

MISSION POINT PRESS

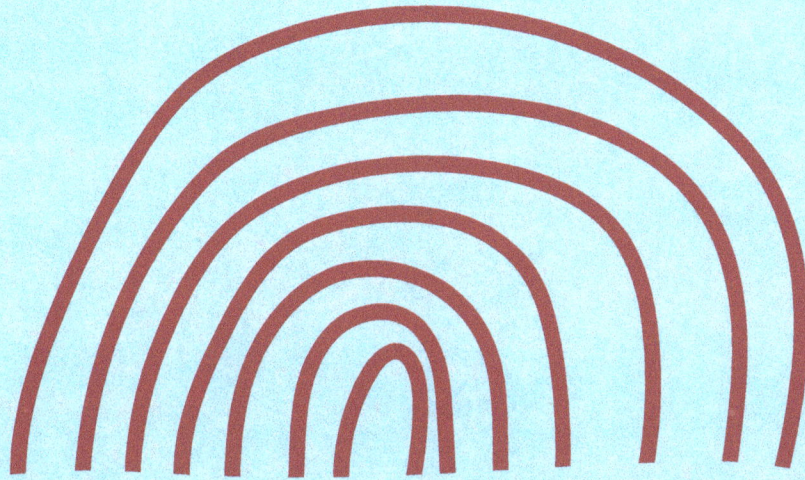

This book is dedicated to my mom who has always supported me. She didn't give up and she didn't let me go.

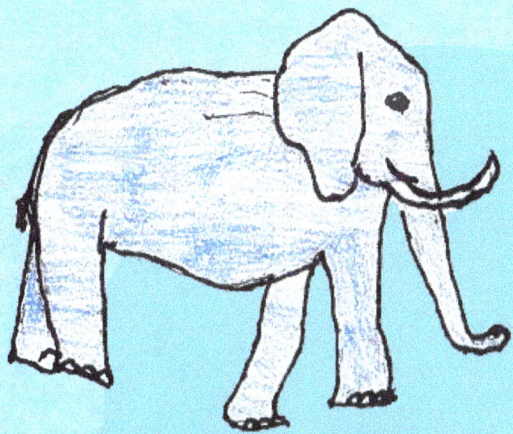

Ami, Emerson's mom, said that when Emerson was first diagnosed she loved elephants. Ami loved how elephants were so protective of their babies and how the herd took care of the young together. Ami and Emerson also watched the Disney movie *Brave* many times, so Ami started calling her "Emerson the Brave."

All proceeds from this book will be donated to the ChadTough Defeat DIPG Foundation to further their research efforts in the hopes of finding a cure.

— EMERSON AND HER FAMILY

Hi, I'm **EMERSON THE BRAVE**, but I wasn't always known as that. My name is Emerson Hoogendoorn. I am 12 years old and I was diagnosed with brain cancer at the age of 6 when I had just finished kindergarten. I had to do many hard and challenging things and I wanted to show kids that it can be scary, but you can do it because I did. In fourth grade, we did a project and wrote ABC books. We all picked a topic and wrote a full cover-to-cover ABC book and mine was things in the hospital. I told my teacher, Ms. Kovacs, that I thought it would be cool to make my little 4th grade project into a real book. I could use it to help kids with cancer and also to make money for my charity.

This book is about my journey with cancer and the hard yet fun and exciting experiences that I've had through it. I wrote this book hoping to inspire kids to be BRAVE and to inform all the kids and even adults how things that happen in the hospital aren't always scary.

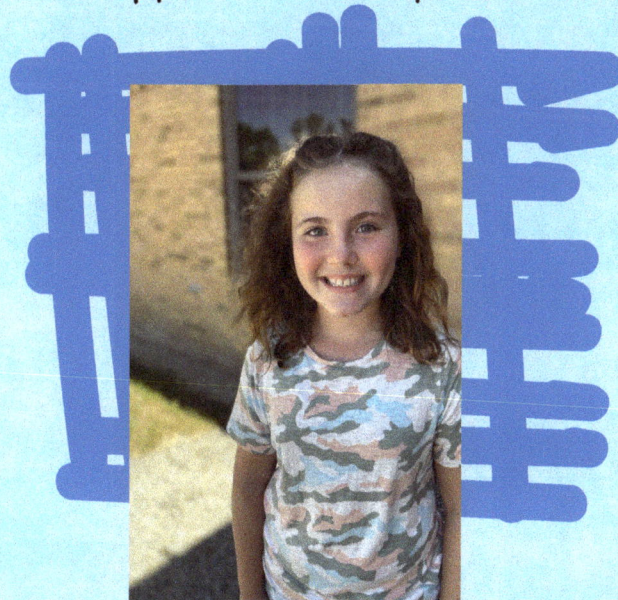

Emerson (4th grade) when she wrote the first draft of her ABC book

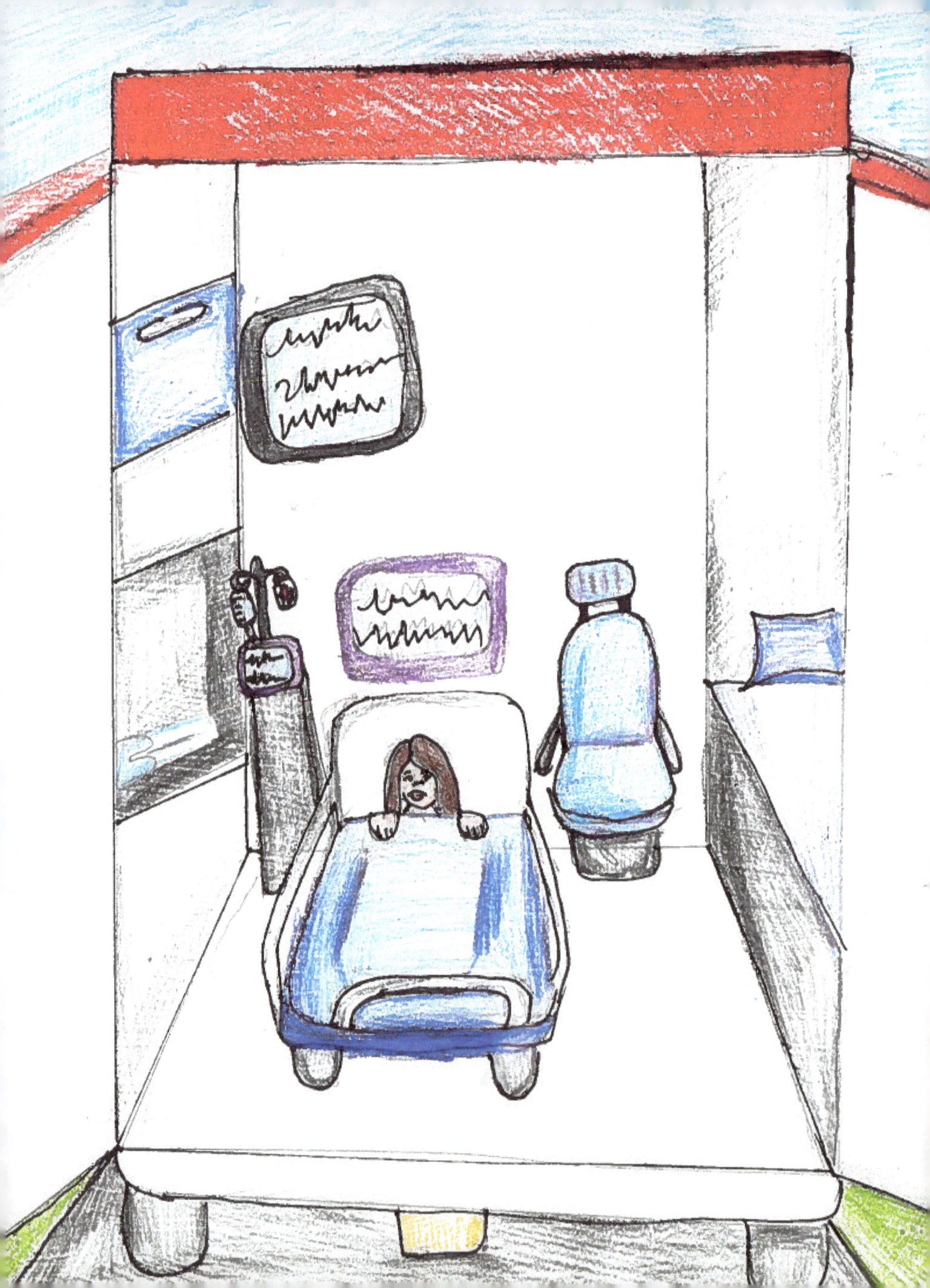

A nxious I felt

M any thoughts in my head

B ouncy ride

U nder bright lights

L ots of medical equipment

A long ride to Grand Rapids

N ot happy

C omfort from my parents

E xtra loud

EMERSON'S STORY

My cancer journey started with a terrible headache. When my mom took me to the emergency room, I had to ride in an ambulance to get from one hospital to the other. The lights were very bright and I got checked on a lot by the paramedics. It was not very pleasant. My mom got to ride with me the whole way to Grand Rapids, with my grandma following the ambulance in her car. Having family with you always helps.

3

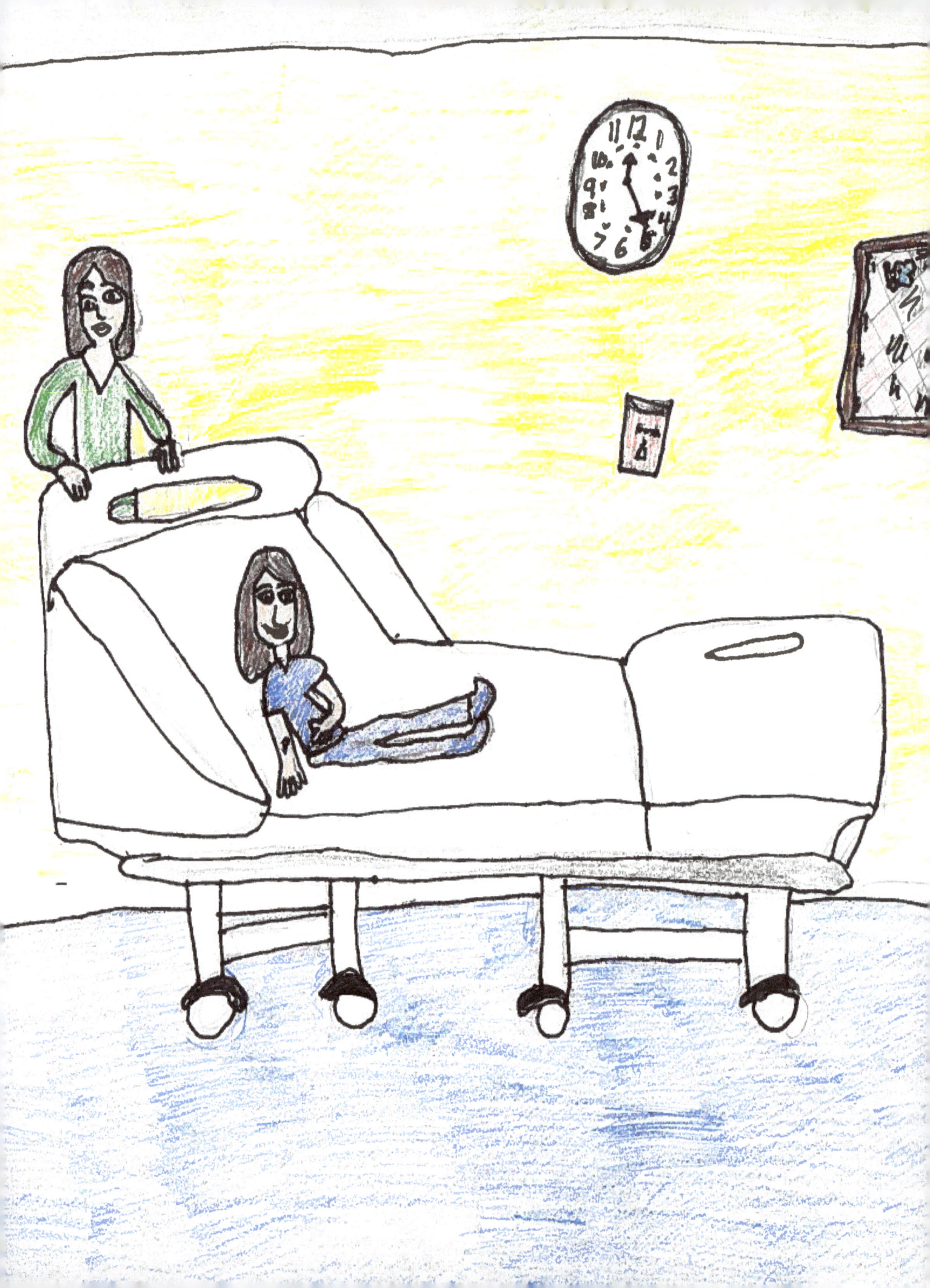

Bumpy ride to my room

Everything was clean

Did not enjoy sleeping in them

B

EMERSON'S STORY

When I was in the hospital, I spent most of my time in bed not doing much. I would lay in the bed and eat and do some fun crafts. Sometimes the Child Life people would come and surprise me with fun things like crafts or toys for me to pick. It was comfy, but not like my bed at home. The only time I got to get up was when I had to go to the bathroom; otherwise, I would just lay in the bed and watch movies. It's okay to ask for snacks!

5

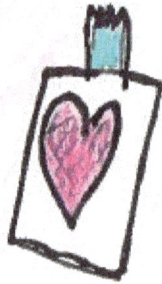

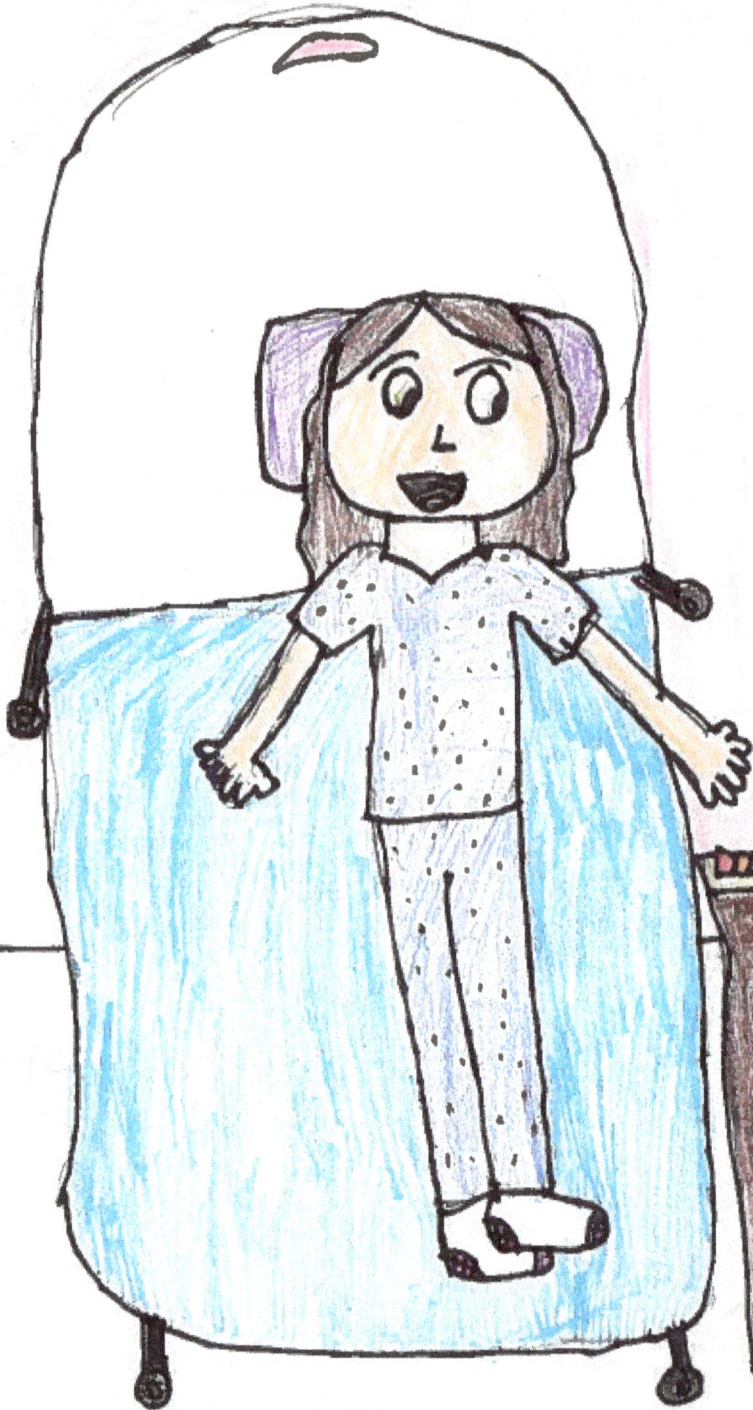

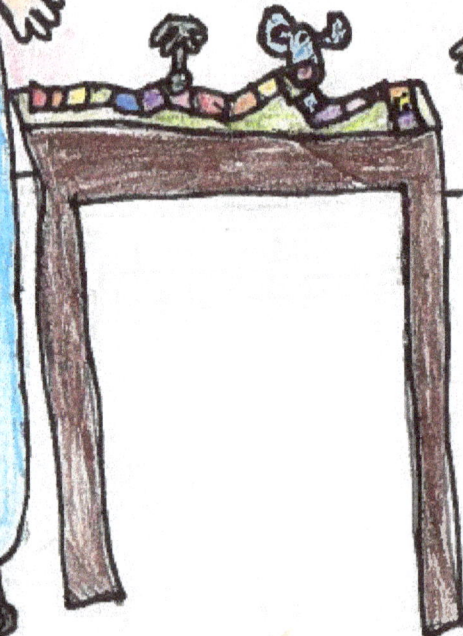

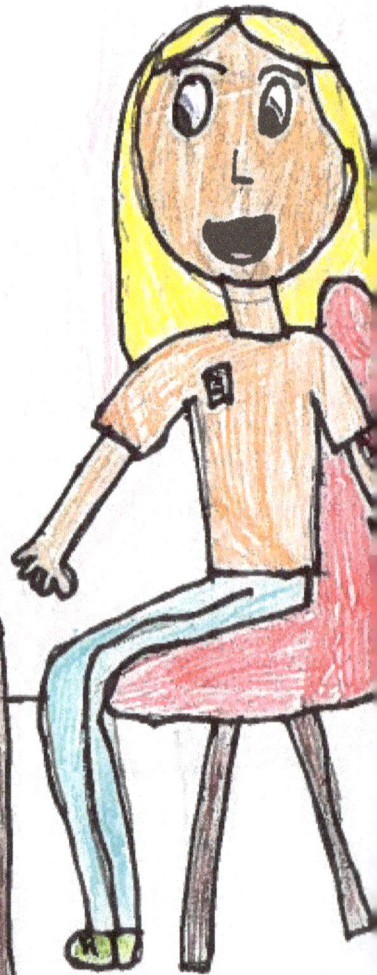

Cheerful and always happy

Helpful when I got my blood drawn

IPads for distraction

Like to have fun

Dedicated to helping kids

Lots of laughs

Informative about MRIs and IVs

Friendly

Excellent support for me

EMERSON'S STORY

Child Life helped me in a lot of different ways, and they are there to help anyone who needs it. One of the ways they helped me was before and after my MRIs, they would come and talk to me. When I was getting my IVs, they would ask me if I had any questions, then they answered them for me. That helped me understand what was about to happen and to make me feel comfortable about it. The Child Life people are there just for kids.

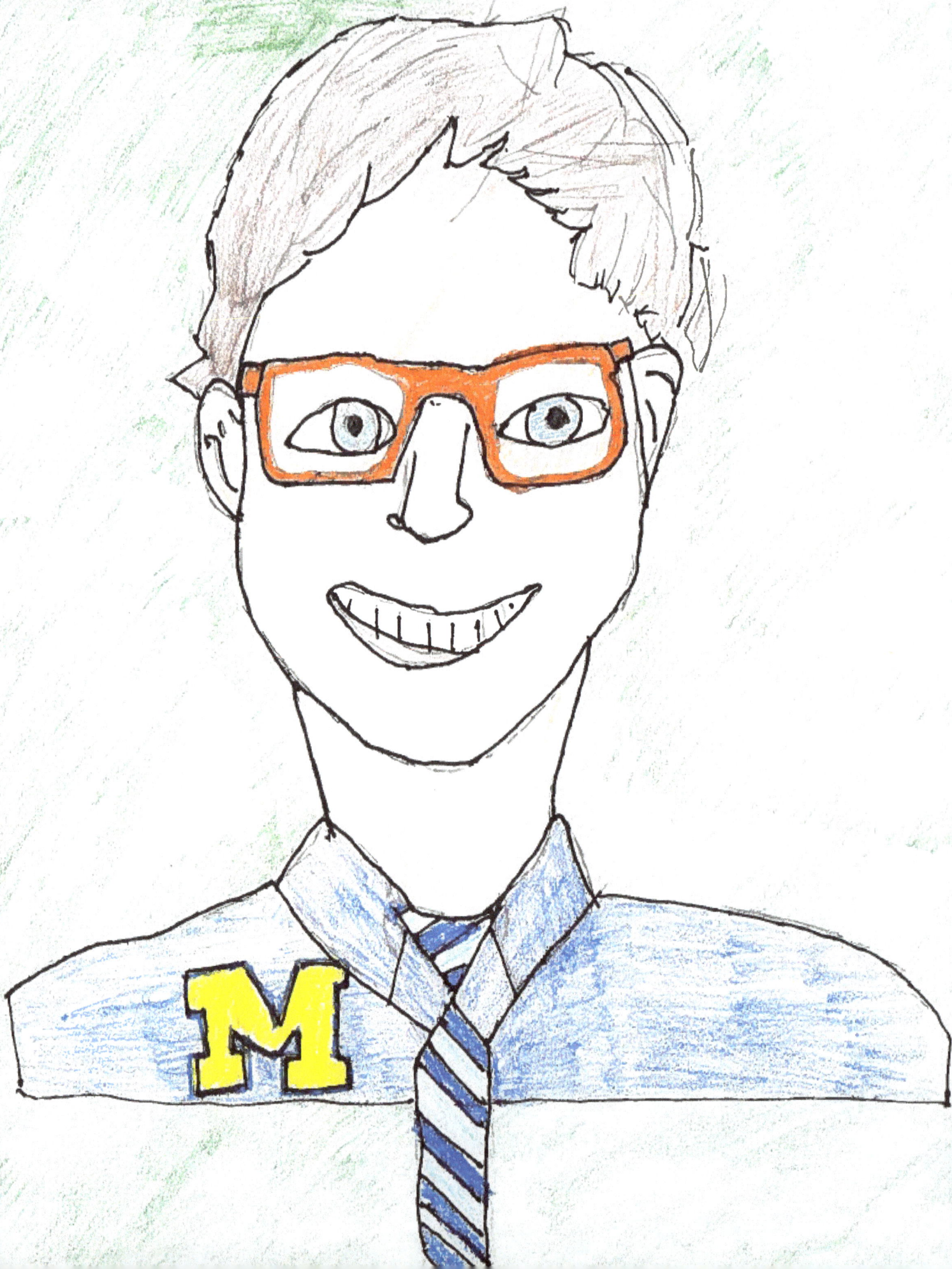

D

Determined to heal kids

Really cool colors (like Blippi!)

Kind

On top of learning new things

Star at the top of the Christmas tree

Compassionate

Hands-on

Medical doctor

Amazing at explaining things to me

No time for dilly-dallying

Never gives up

EMERSON'S STORY

Dr. Koschmann is many things to me. He is the doctor in Ann Arbor that takes care of me and monitors my cancer. He also is a researcher; he collects information from my blood and my scans and uses that to learn more about cancer and how to make new treatments for other kids with or without the same kind of tumor. He is my favorite doctor and has been with me for my entire journey. Every kid needs someone like Dr. Koschmann.

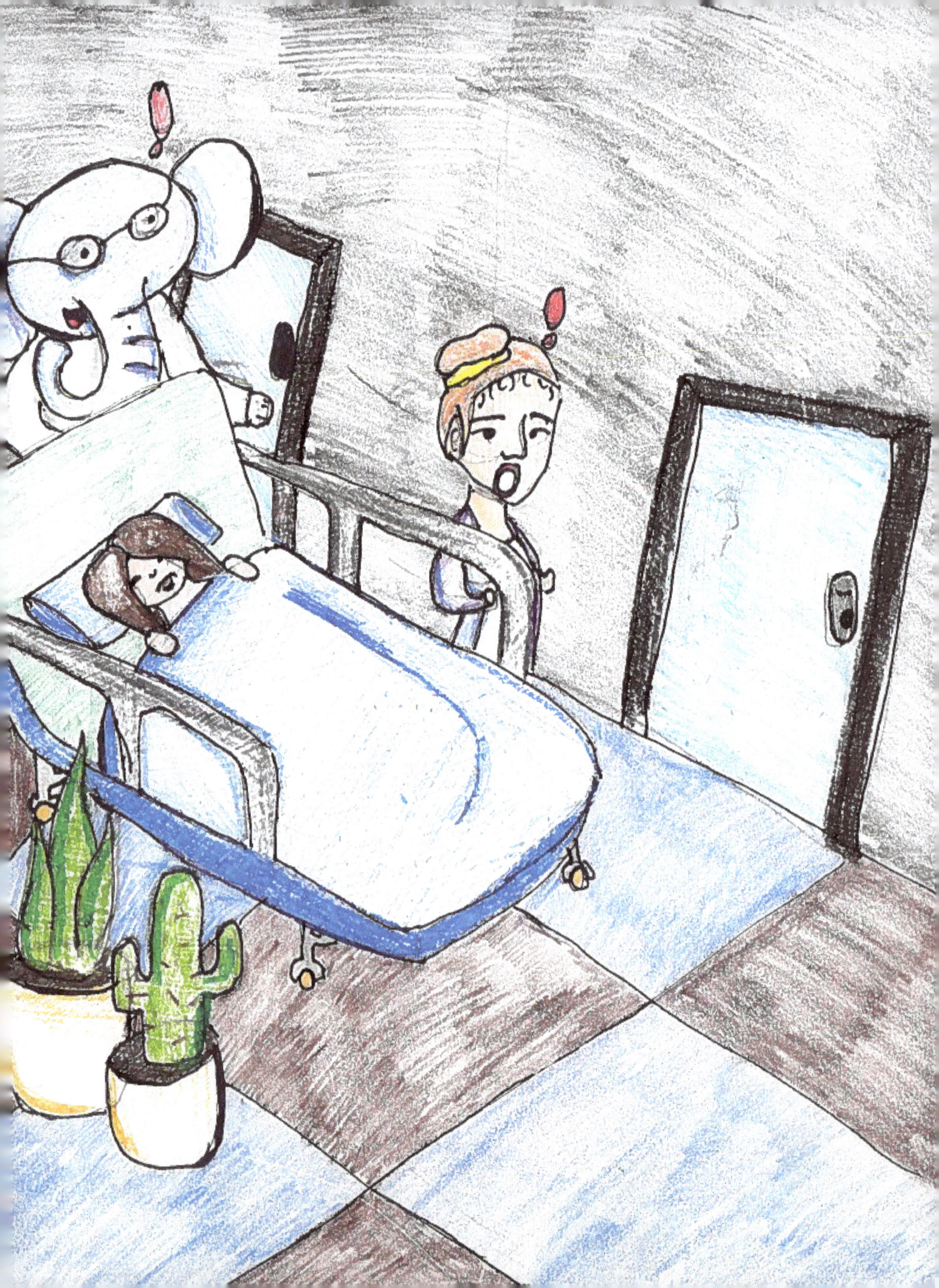

Extreme emotions

Mom was there beside me

Entertained in my bed

Really intense

Guests at the hospital

Everybody had to move fast

Nervously waiting for my results

Caution signs everywhere

Yield — sharp things, don't touch!

EMERSON'S STORY

The Emergency Room is a special place at the hospital where people take care of you when something unexpected happens. I went through the emergency entrance at the hospital at the end of my first ambulance ride, and I had so much pain in my head that it was considered an emergency. That's when I knew that my cancer journey had started. I'm glad they were there to help.

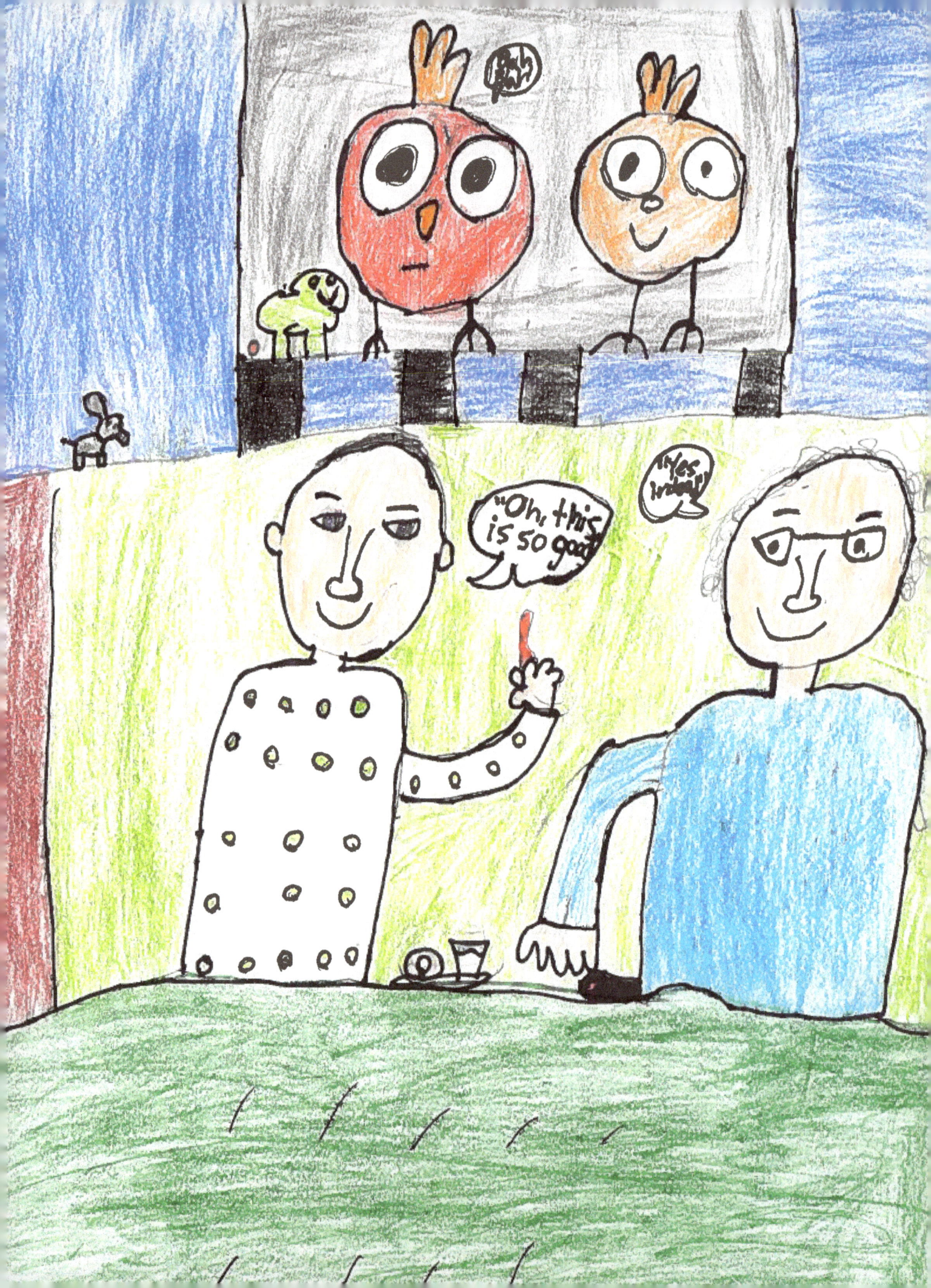

Free for patients

Oooooh, it was so good!

Organic and fresh

Doughnuts and milk

F

EMERSON'S STORY

There was a lot of great food at the hospital. One of my favorite foods was their sausage, and my grandma would eat it together with me in my bed. We could also order food and one of my favorites was Buffalo Wild Wings. I remember that I drank all the apple juice that they had on my floor. I would also love to eat Nacho Cheese Doritos. You can ask for foods you like.

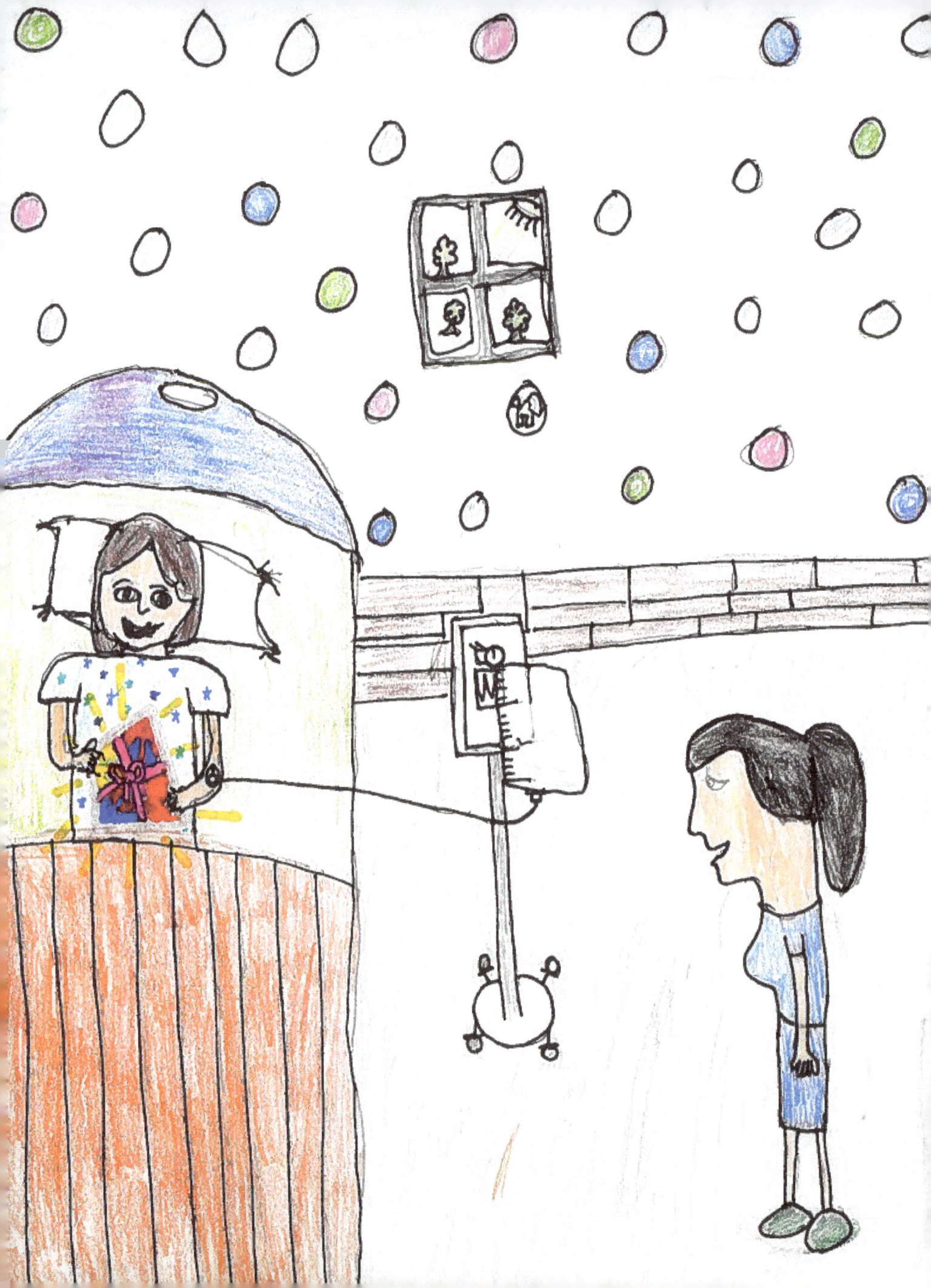

Gifts from family and friends

I felt grateful

Fluffy stuffed elephant

Tons of LEGOs

Surprised by all my visitors!

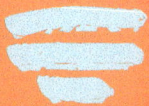

G

EMERSON'S STORY

I got a ton of visits from my friends and family members when I was in the hospital, and they often brought gifts like stuffed animals, crafts, LEGOs, and slime. All things to keep me busy and entertained while being in the hospital. Kids like to know their friends are thinking of them when they're sick.

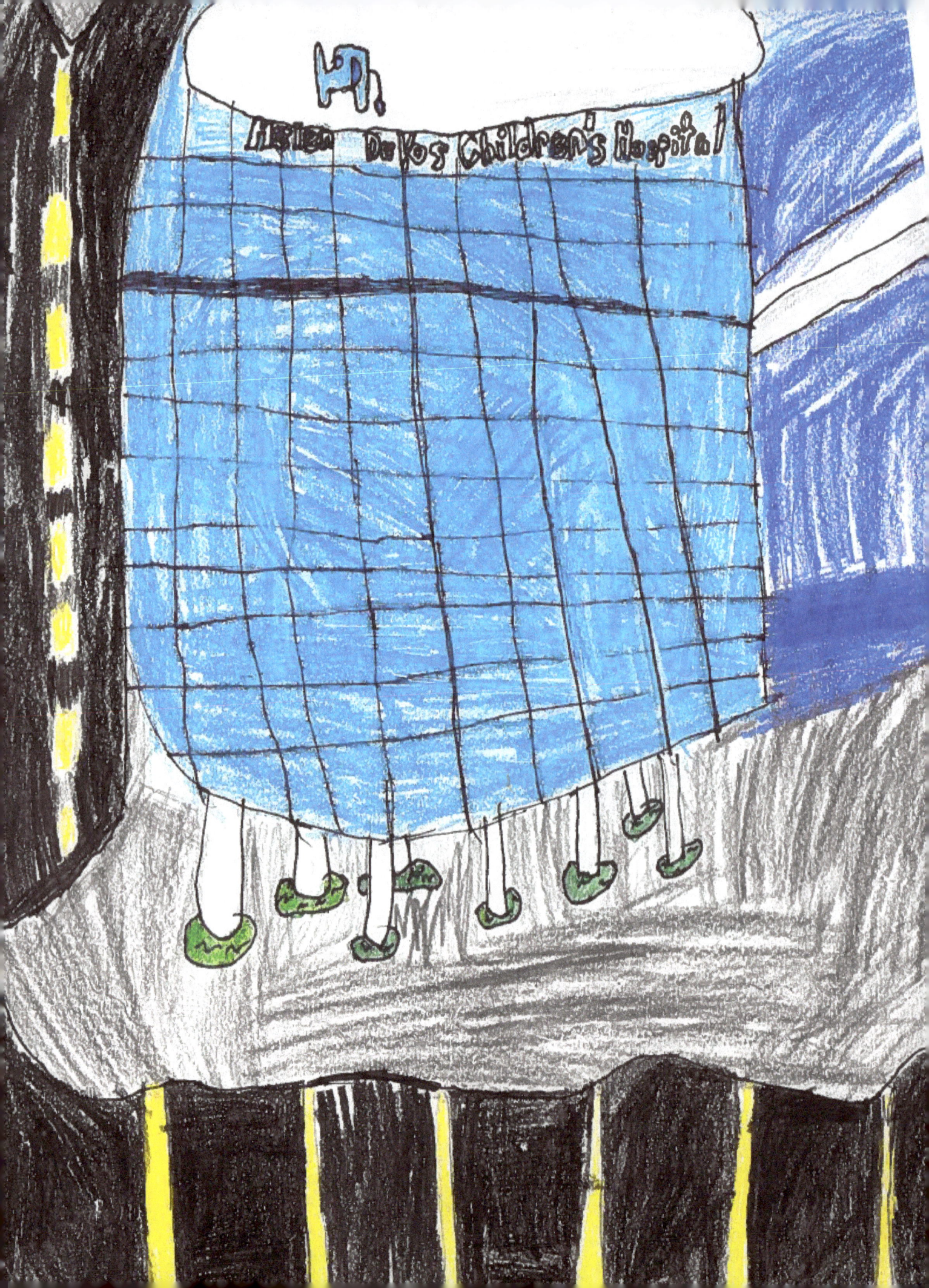

Heat pads for my IVs

Elevators to many floors

Laboratory where I get my labs done

Excellent care from the nurses

Nighttime sirens I could hear

Delivered food and drinks

Everyone gets a clean room

Very happy place

Operations on my brain

Stayed there for 11 days

EMERSON'S STORY

Helen DeVos Children's Hospital is in Grand Rapids, Michigan. It is where the ambulance took me to after they found the tumor in my brain at Holland Hospital. I had surgery on my brain to remove part of the tumor at Helen DeVos. This is also where I go for some of my follow-up care. They take care of a lot of kids who are sick.

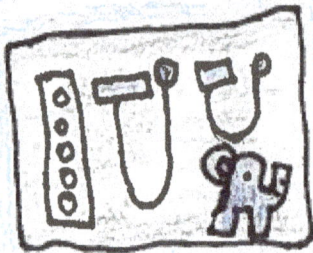

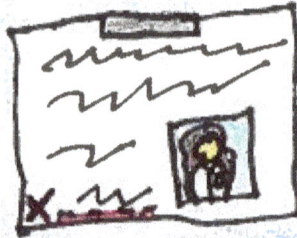

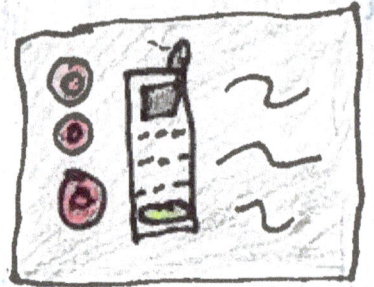

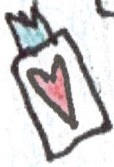

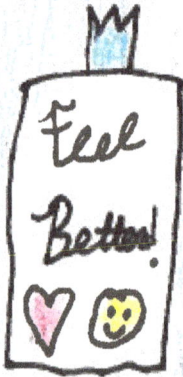

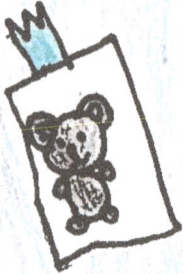

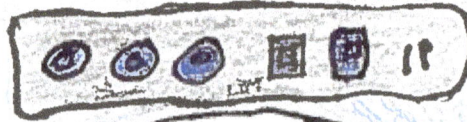

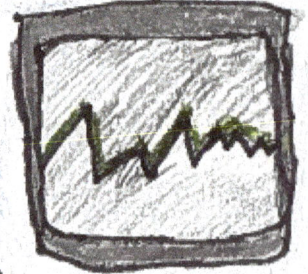

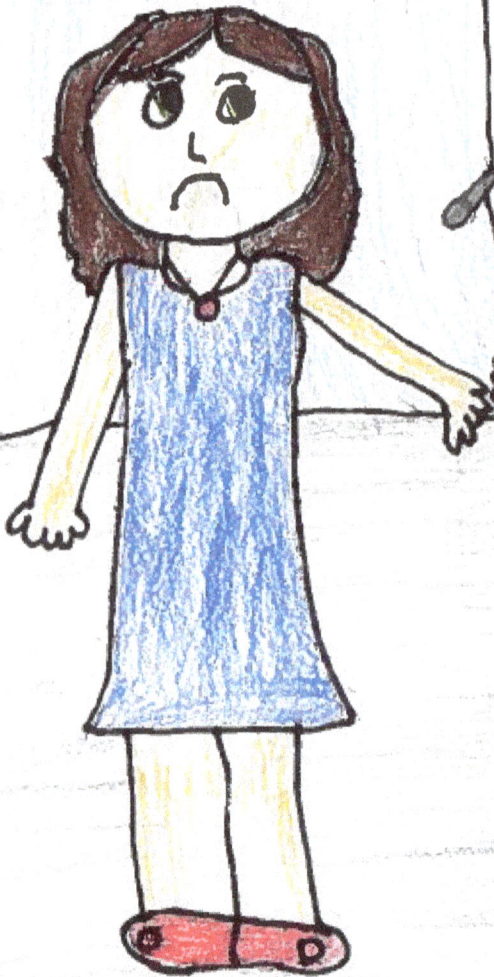

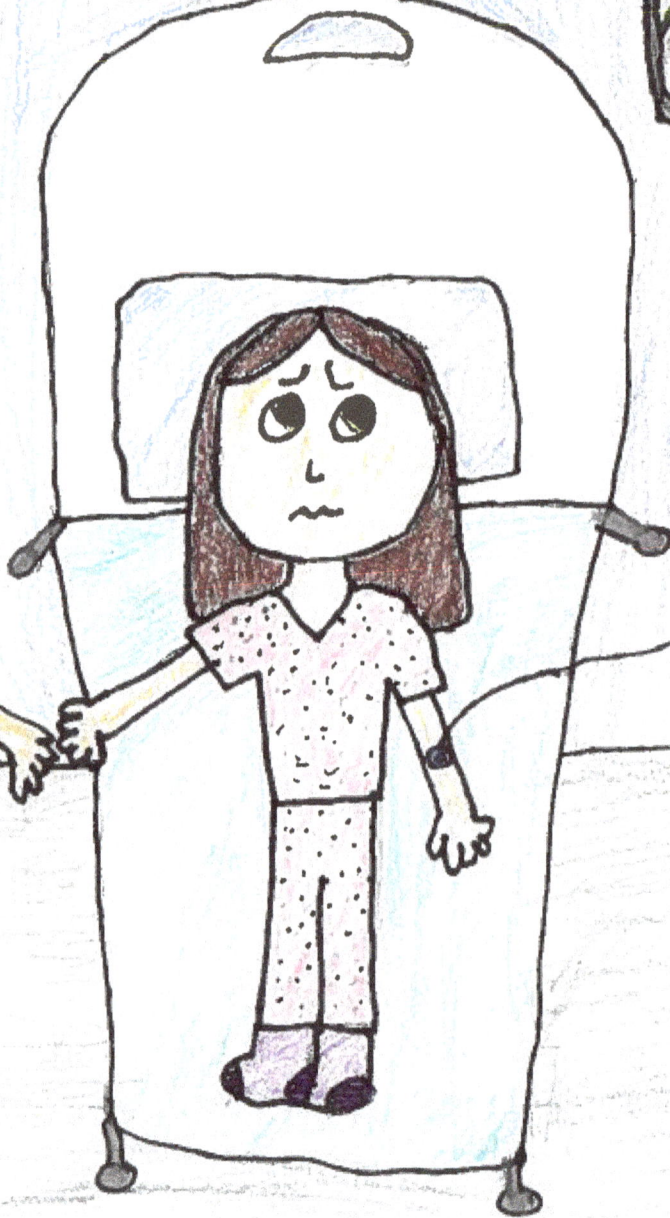

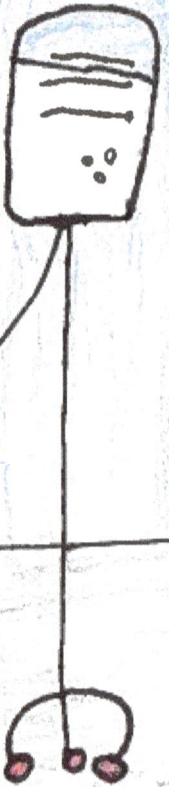

Intensive is for people
    who need lots of attention

Care is what they give you

United hospital staff

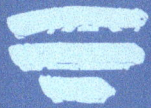

ICU stands for Intensive Care Unit, which is where I went after my two surgeries. My nurses and doctors were there, and my parents were there with me, too. I stayed there just after my surgery to make sure that my body was working properly after my huge brain surgery. They take really good care of you.

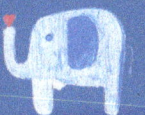

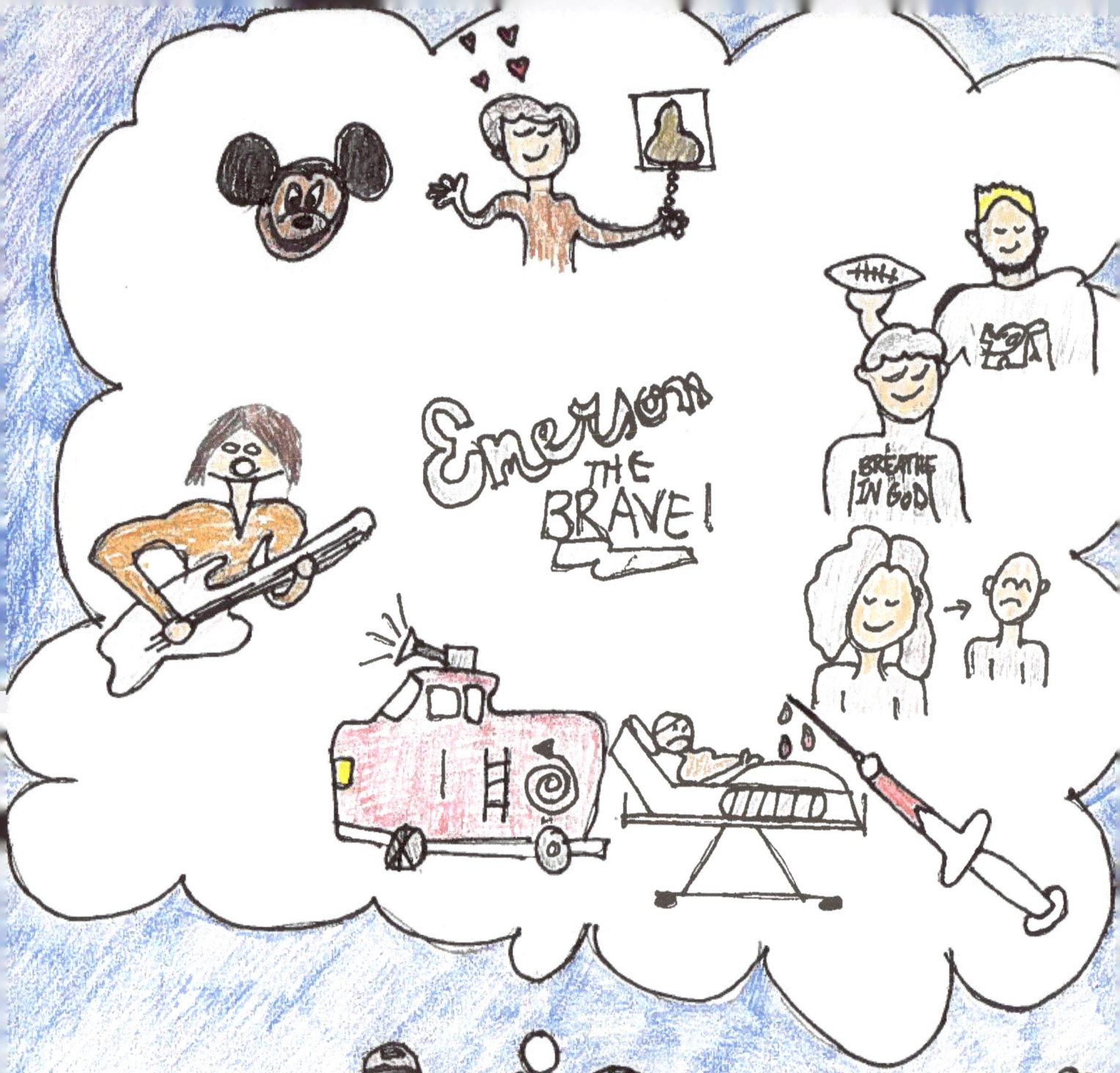
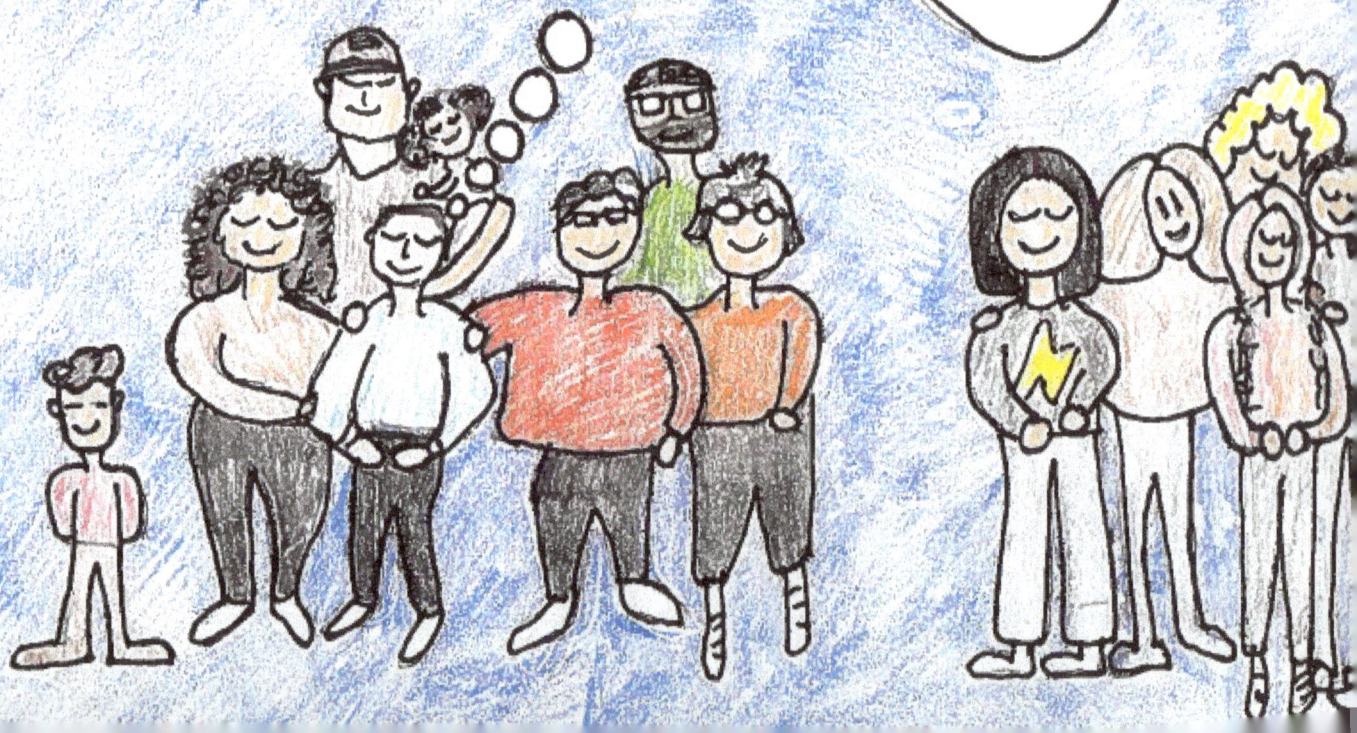

Just made it through treatment

On a new medication

Under lots of pressure

Radiation to shrink my tumor

New things take place every day

Empathy for other kids

Yesterday I was Emerson…
today I'm **EMERSON THE BRAVE**

EMERSON'S STORY

After all the surgeries and radiation and chemotherapy, I started on my new experimental drug, ONC201. It was supposed to fight my bad cancer cells and add to my good ones. It helped me feel like me again. I hope all kids with cancer have a chance for a treatment.

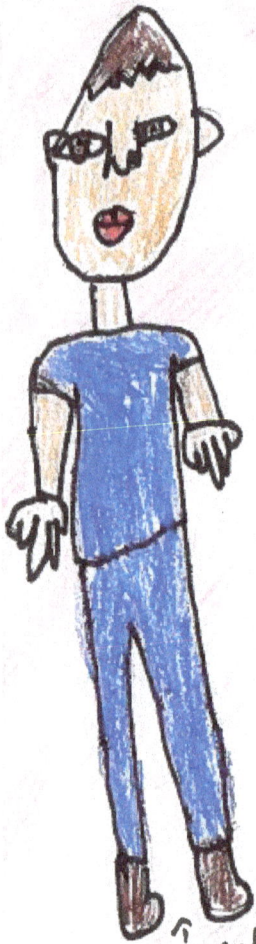

Dr Koshmann

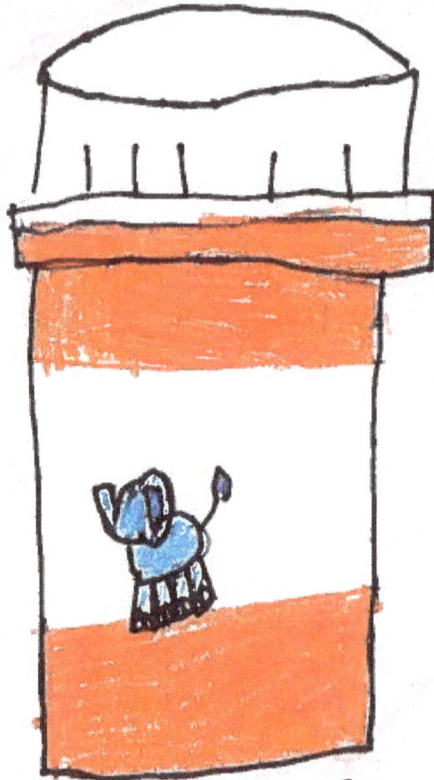

Onc 201

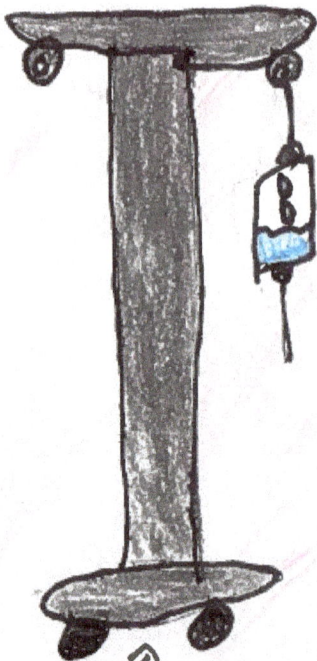

IV

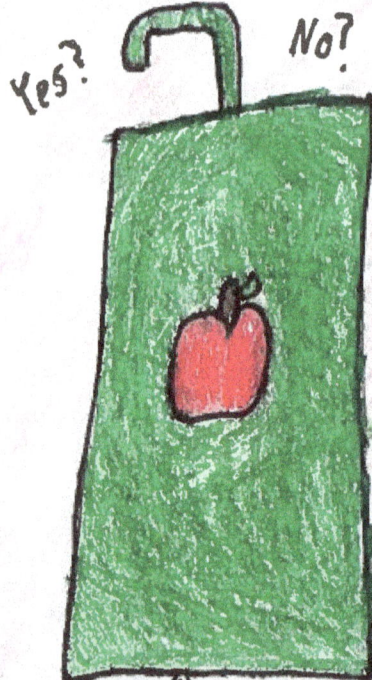

Yes?   No?

Aaple "Juice"

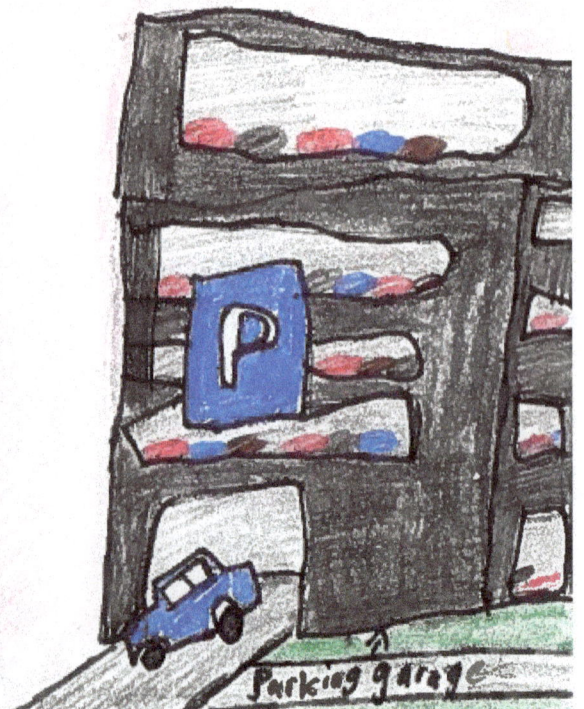

Parking garage

Koschmann is my researcher

No one fights alone

Onc201 — my experimental meds

When to drink apple juice after IVs

Learning my own strength

Experiencing some scary times

Donating to spread awareness

Getting the MRI bed set up

Entering the parking garage and finding a parking spot

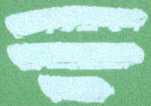

EMERSON'S STORY

My family and I have learned a lot of things we didn't know before I had cancer. My doctors and nurses know all kinds of techniques that help me get through all kinds of procedures, like "Buzzy the Bee" that helps when you get IVs. I'm glad I know a lot about cancer treatments, but sometimes I wish I didn't have to.

23

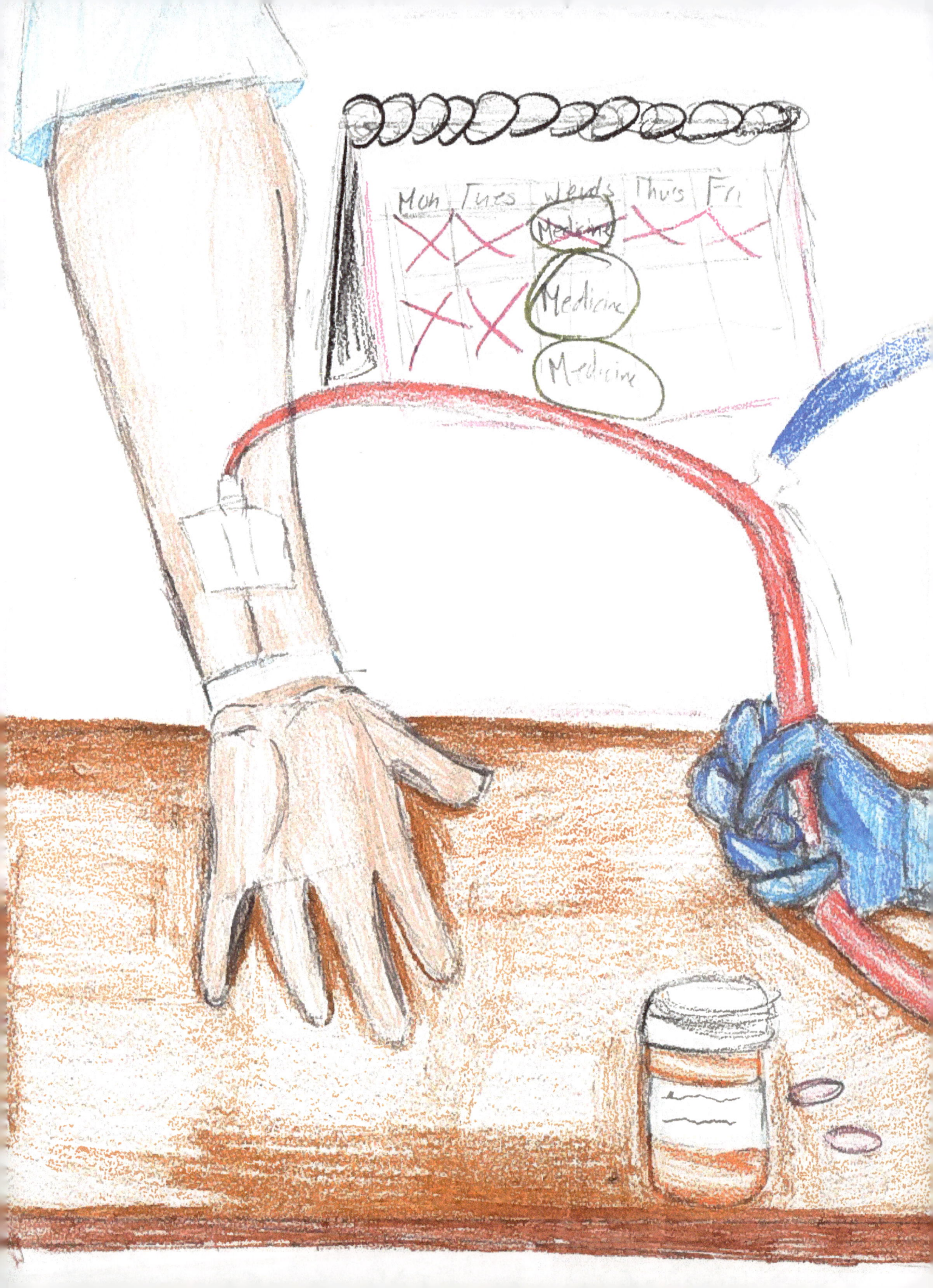

Labs drawn on my arms

Antibiotics — five every Wednesday

Blood…you get used to it

One quick poke

Radiation treatments

A way to get information

Tests on my blood on every visit

Oncology floor

Rubber gloves to keep safe

Your techs are helpful

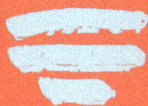

EMERSON'S STORY

Every three weeks, I would go to Grand Rapids for blood draws and checkups, and every nine weeks I'd go to Ann Arbor for MRIs. It was a lot of appointments, but I kind of got used to it after a while. Without labs, we wouldn't know if the experimental drug was doing its job. I used to wonder why I had to get poked so often, and my mom and grandma would say, "It's to make sure your blood is healthy." Labs are important!

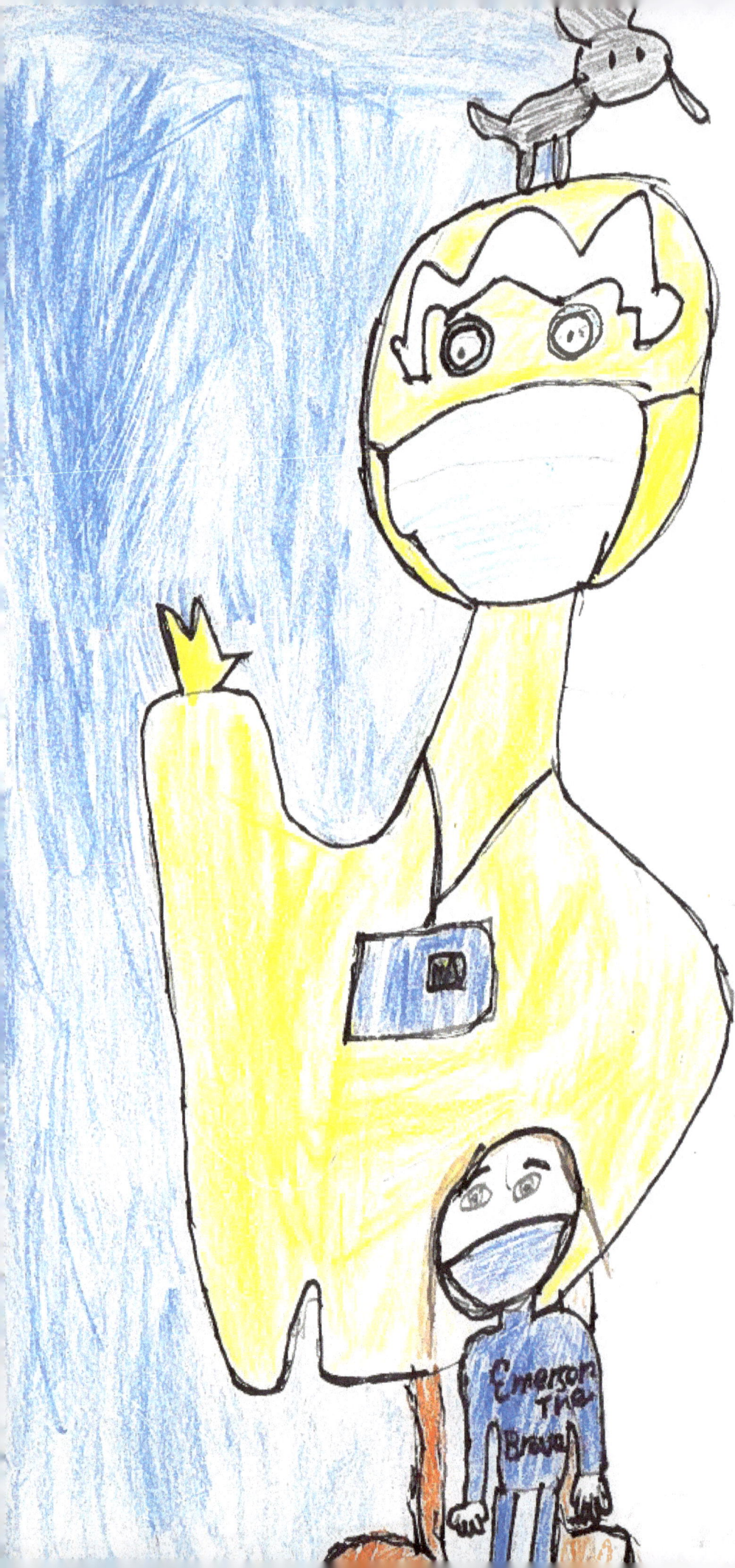

Emerson
The
Brave

Moving on a table

Really noisy

Inside a tube you go

EMERSON'S STORY

MRI means Magnetic Resonance Imaging, which is kind of like an x-ray where they can see inside your body. When I get an MRI, I lay on a bed while they get me all situated. The bed moves inside a tube, and I'm not supposed to move. The machine is super-duper loud. They usually put a mirror inside so I can see my grandma's face and watch a movie. That helps. Sometimes it can take up to an hour. Kids need to be sure and tell someone if they are scared.

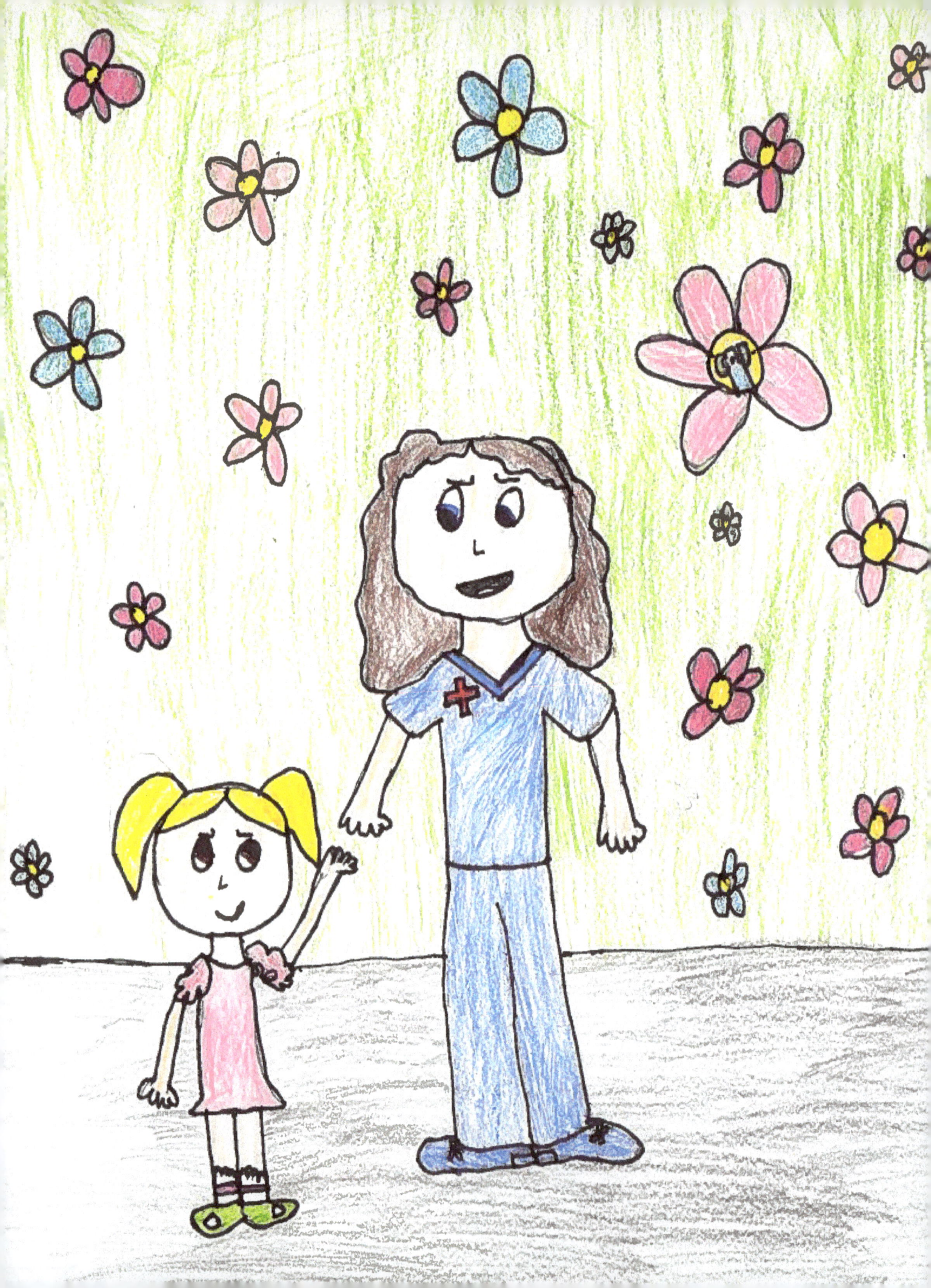

Never-ending care

Understanding to everyone

Ready for the unexpected

Super explainable to me

Excited and hyped up

So kind

EMERSON'S STORY

I love all the nurses. Nurses are there to help YOU so you have to tell them what you need so they can do their job and help you. They are very kind, they explain things, they help you. They keep an eye on things, check your blood pressure, and help you go to the bathroom. One time when I couldn't even walk, my nurse carried me to the toilet at the side of my bed. The nurses are with you all the time.

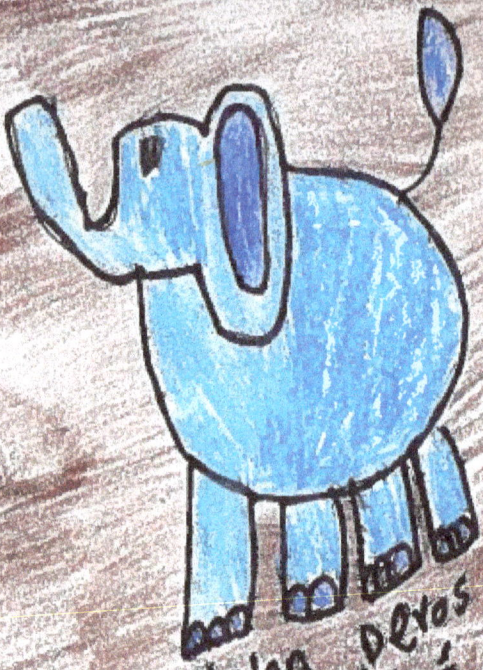

Helen Devos
Children's Hospital

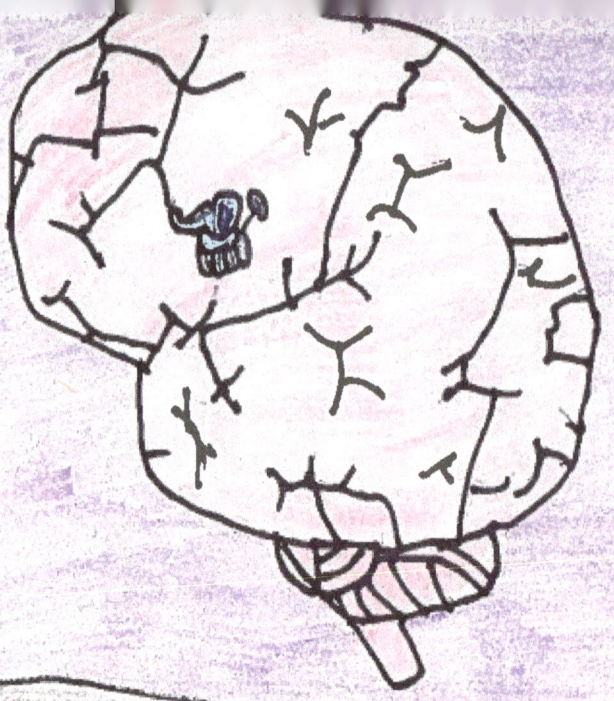

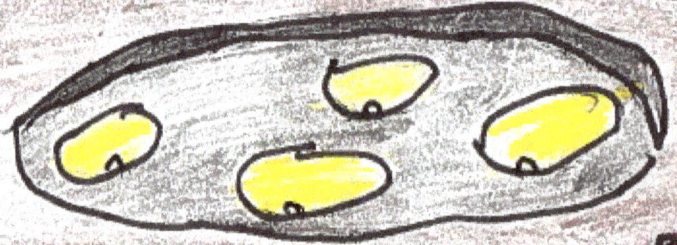

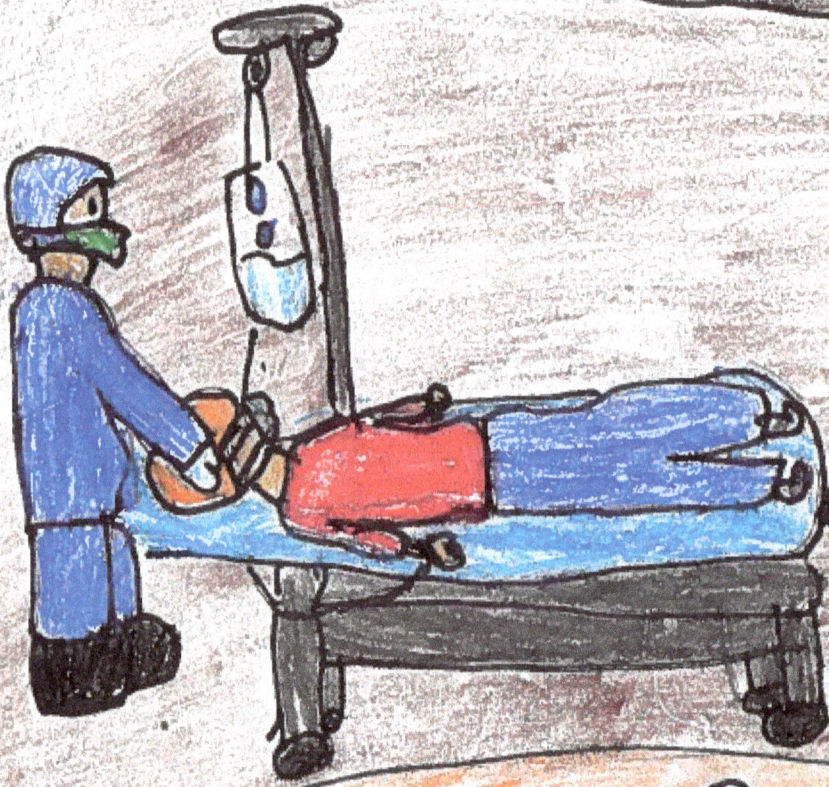

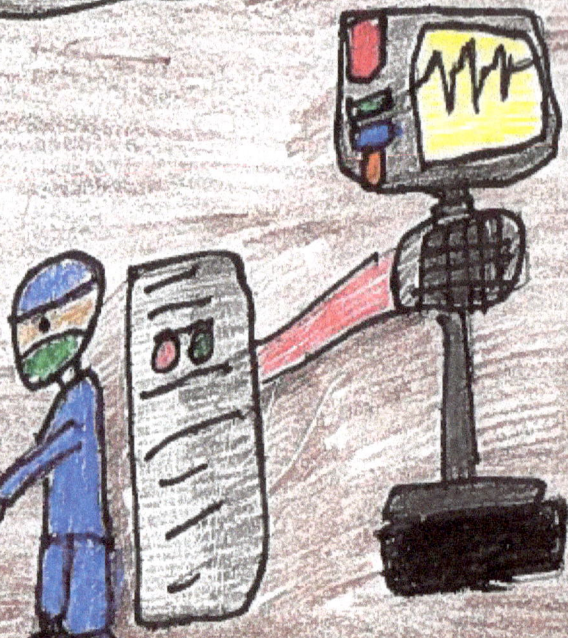

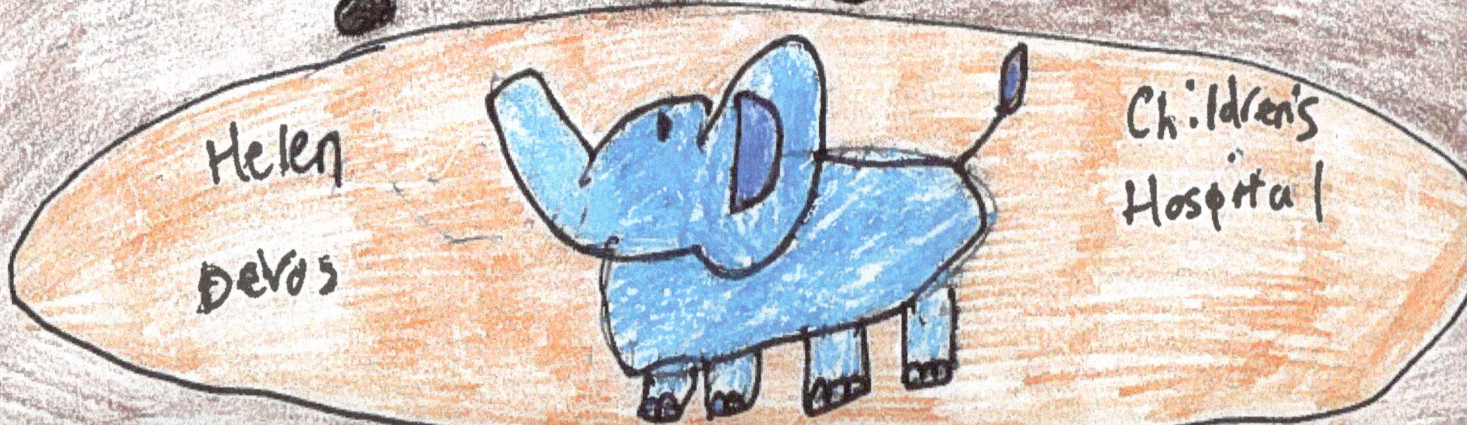

Helen
Devos

Children's
Hospital

Operation on my brain

Photos of my brain in my surgery

Entering the operating room

Really scary

Anesthesia put me asleep

Toes in socks

Iv in my arm to keep me sedated

Opening my eyes in recovery

Not feeling a single thing

EMERSON'S STORY

I had two operations when I was in first grade. They took out most of my brain tumor. I remember myself doing the dab. Sometimes I'd be really happy and sometimes I'd be really upset about something. When I was constipated (which often happens after surgery), I used to sit on the toilet and play Bunny Pop on my grandma's phone. At the hospital, pooping is a good thing! My doctor Mary always said, "bowels and urine," but I always say poop and pee. You get used to these things.

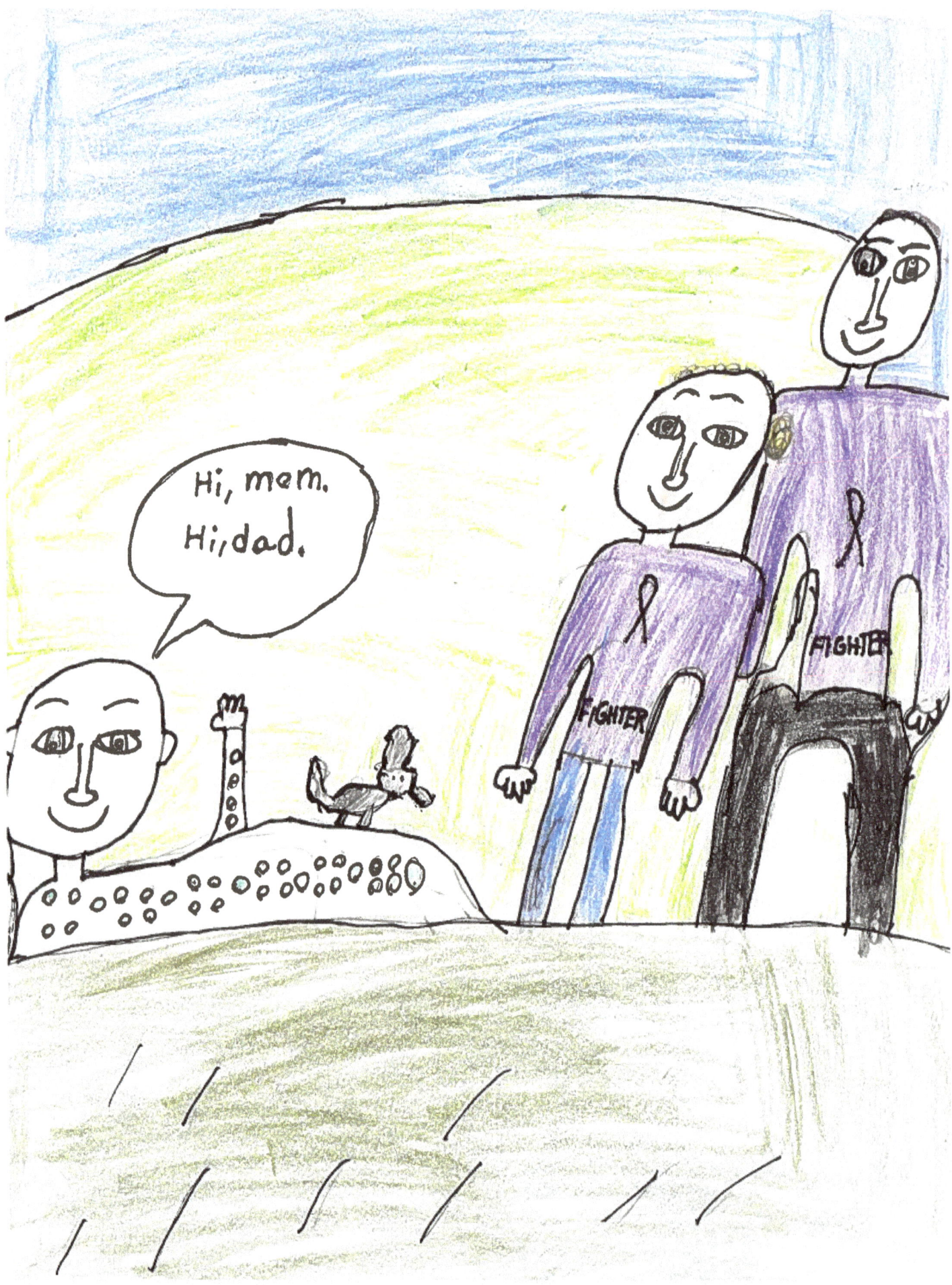

Patiently waiting for me to wake up

Anxious for me

Really loving and caring

Every second having more hope

Never letting me go

They gave their everything

Supported me on my journey

EMERSON'S STORY

My parents have been very supportive since I first got cancer, and also my grandparents. They are the ones who said they weren't going to let me die. They saved my life by finding the experimental treatment that's keeping me stable. My family has been on my journey with me the whole way. Without them, I wouldn't be here.

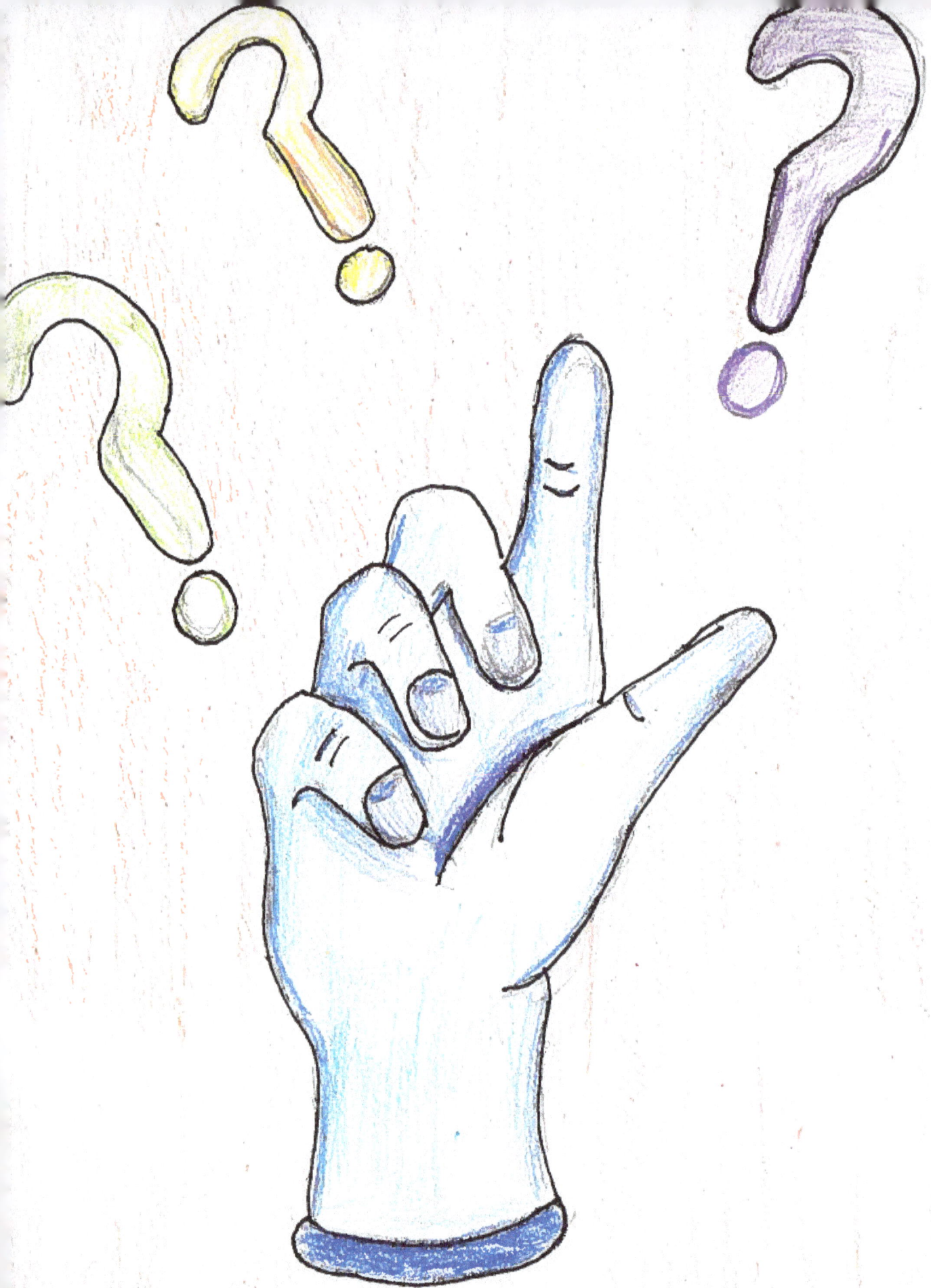

Quick results and answers

Unexpected news can come at any time

Everyone asks them

Sometimes answers can be scary

The doctors are really helpful

It's a good thing to ask questions

On surgery day, I asked many!

Nurses helped too

Sometimes answers are good

EMERSON'S STORY

I have had a lot of questions. And so have my parents and my grandparents. It's okay to ask questions. Sometimes, doctors would ask, "Do you have any questions?" and I would automatically say, "No." I have learned to ask questions. I could always ask my mom or my grandma a question about everything. Kids should talk to their families when they need answers to their questions.

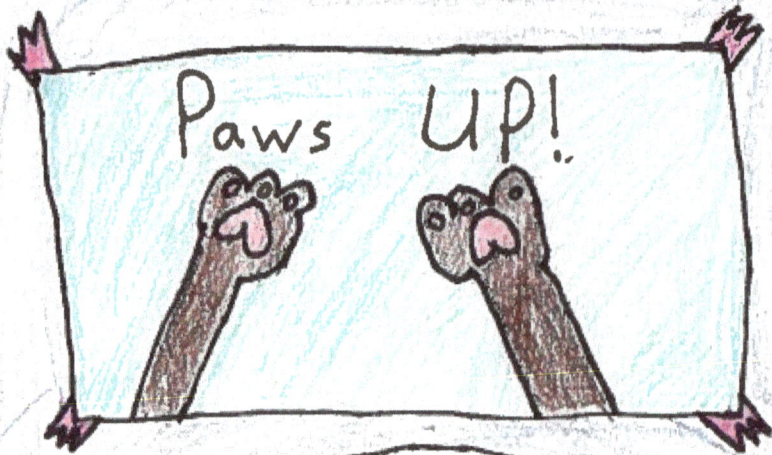

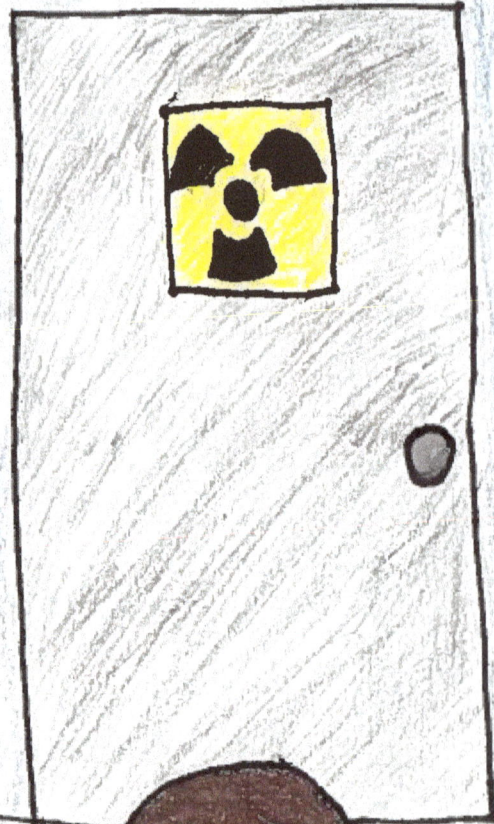

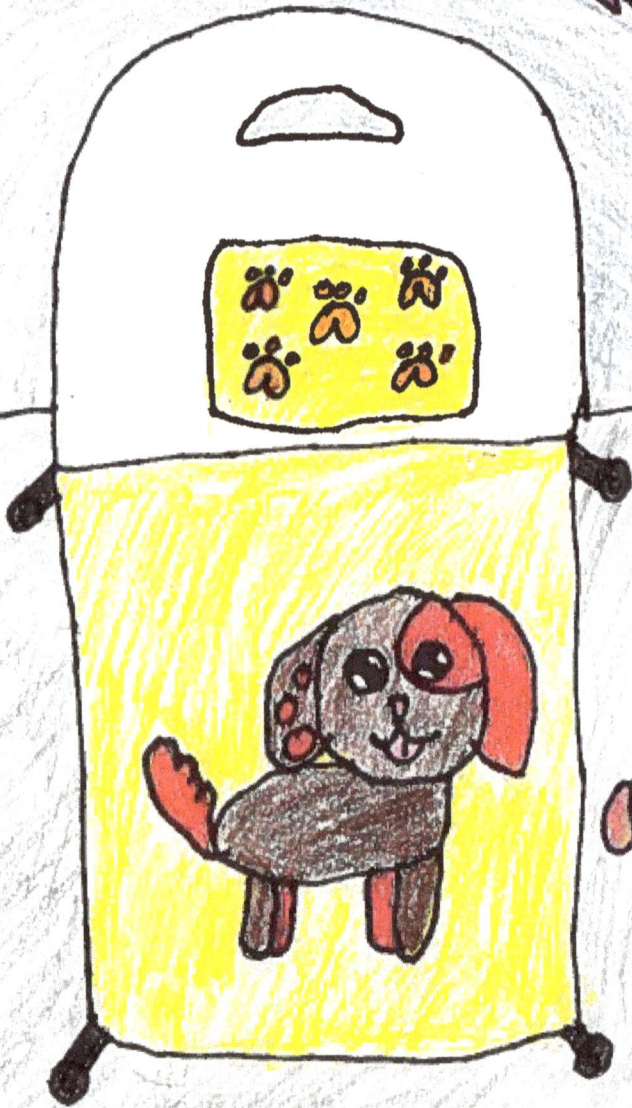

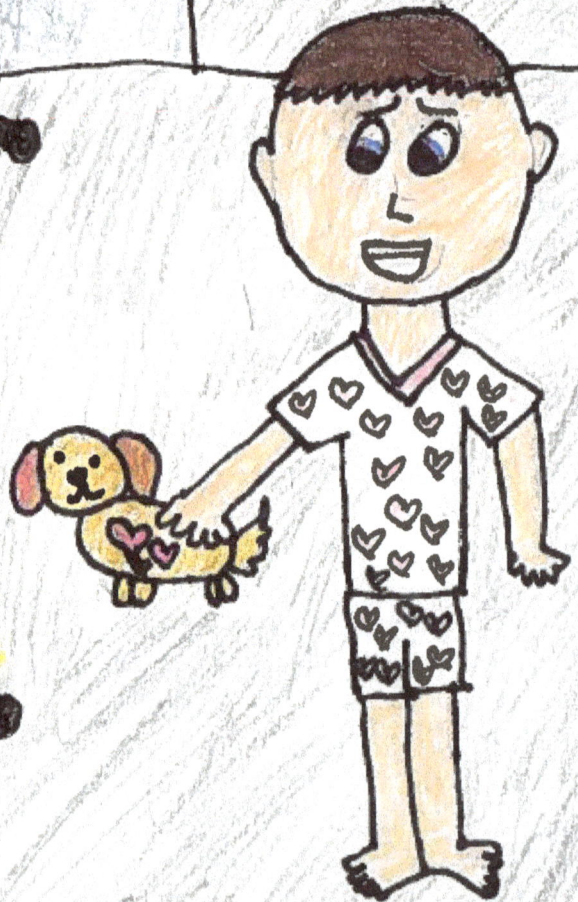

Ready for treatment

Appointments every day

Determined to finish

It can get intense

A challenge to get through

The snuggly stuffed animals helped

I did not like it very much

On my way to being cancer free

K**N**ots in my stomach before the scan

EMERSON'S STORY

The hardest part about radiation is I lost my hair. My grandma and mom cut it off in their kitchen. My dad and my uncle let me buzz their hair off in the driveway. I found a saying that said, "Bald is beautiful, no hair don't care!" My hair grew back pretty fast. Some people looked at me a little weird, and I've been called a boy. But most people act like, "no hair don't care!"

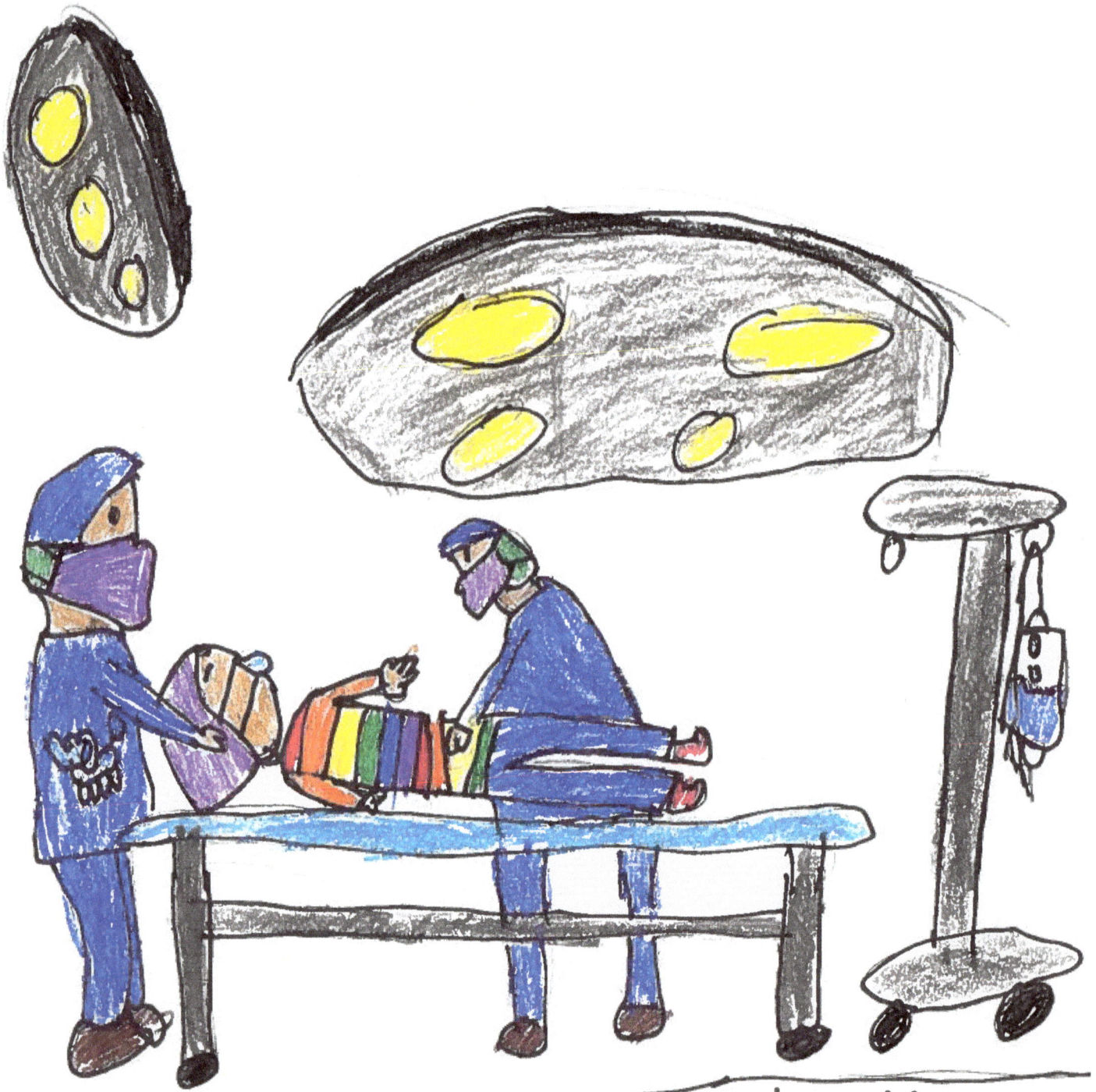

Spectrum Health

Helen DeVos

Children's hospital

Saying goodbye to my family

Under anesthesia

Ready to be done

Getting more wiggly

Excellent care

Really warm when I woke up

Yet another treatment

EMERSON'S STORY

Before the surgery, I was hungry because I couldn't eat for two days. They gave me a flavored tongue depressor. I said goodbye to my mom and they wheeled me back into the room. My surgery happened overnight and I woke up in the morning when it was light. You don't even know it's happening. You go to sleep, wake up, and it's over. You're sore, but it's done. Everyone was there to help.

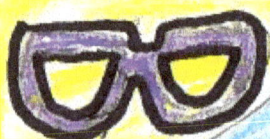

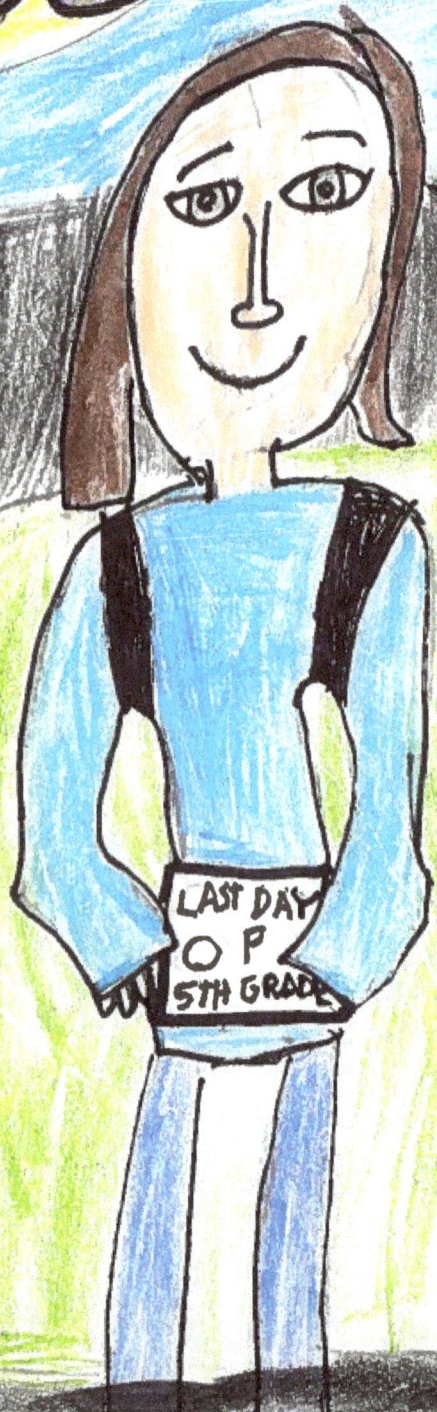

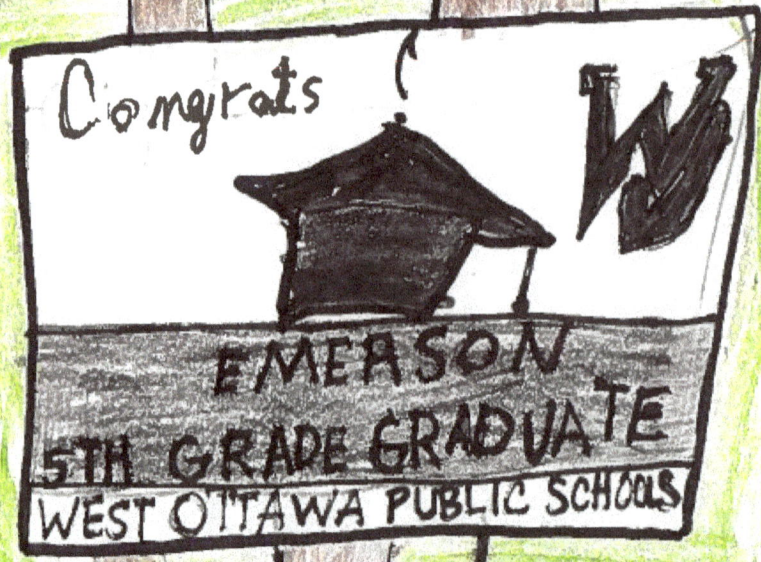

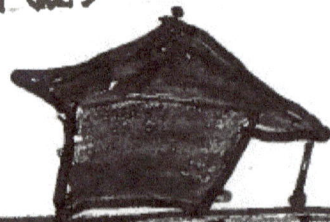

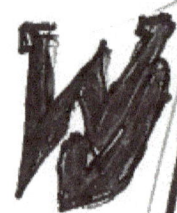

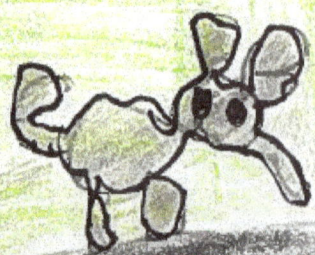

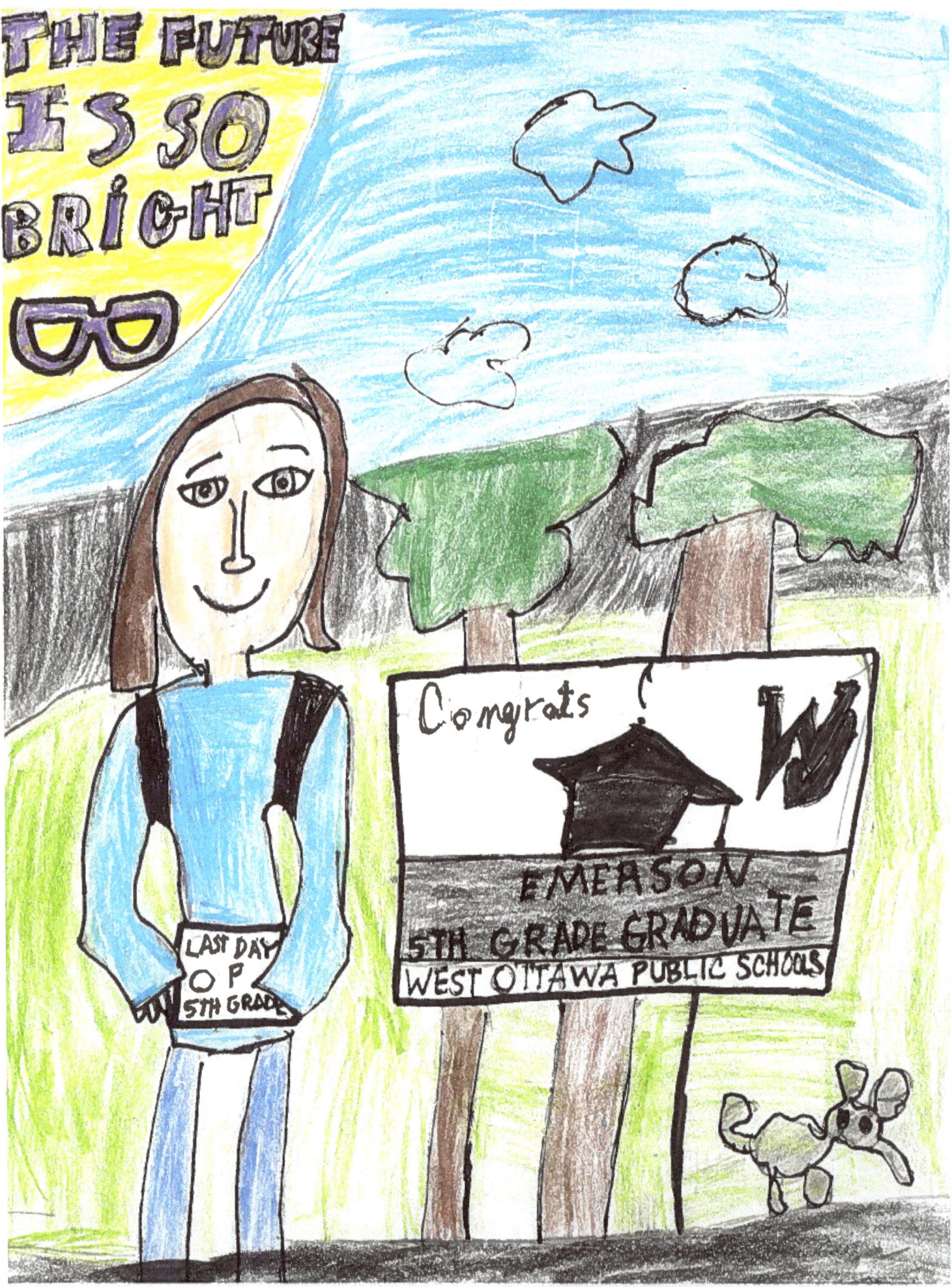

The future is now

On to new plans

Doing things I've looked forward to

A long way I've come

Yet more in my future!

EMERSON'S STORY

When I finished, Child Life gave me a stuffed dog and a prize box to bring home. I got to ring the bell and everyone came out of their room to clap for me. I also made a journey necklace, and each bead meant something for my whole entire cancer life — 50 clear beads for radiation, birthdays, lost a tooth, blood draws — each bead is different. It's still hanging in my room. I looked most forward to swimming and playing with my friends, going to birthday parties, and being in school. I learned to appreciate everyday things.

Be Brave

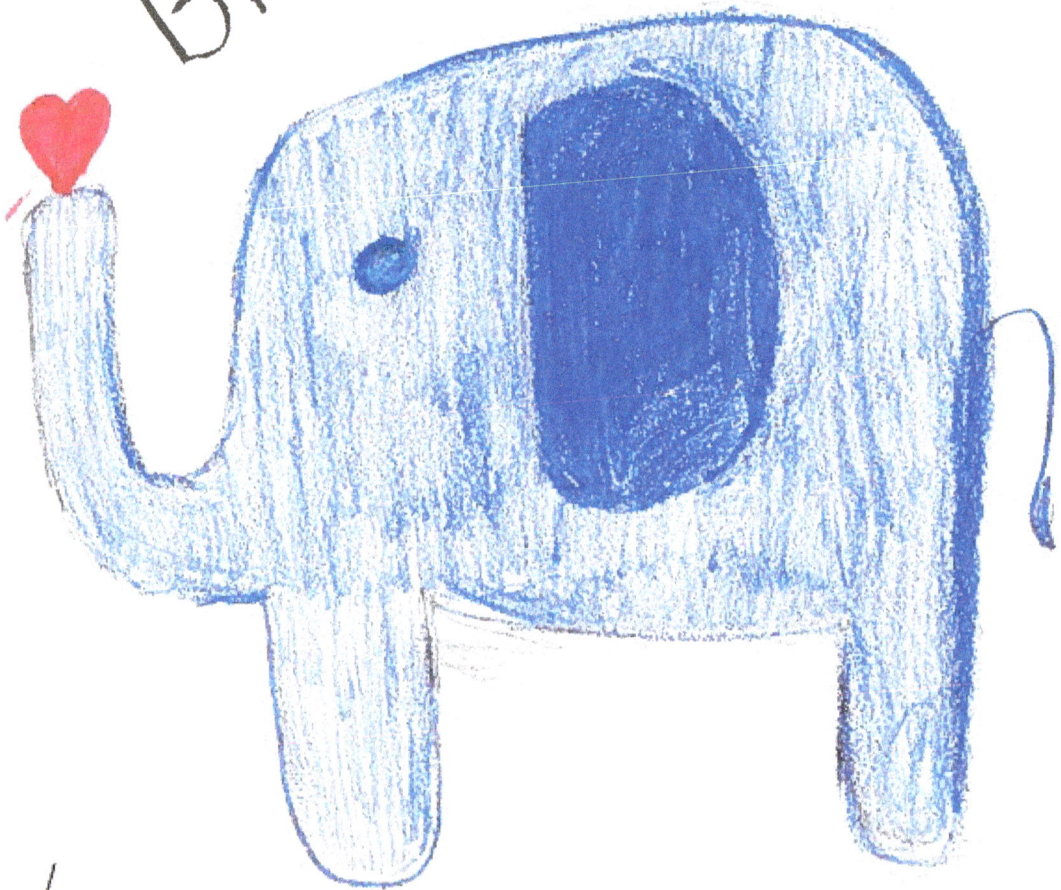

Emerson the Brave

Unbelievable results

Never stop believing

I'm fighting cancer;
  what's your superpower?

Quitting is not an option

Unique in my own way

Everything happens for a reason

EMERSON'S STORY

I was hoping to make this more about the reader than myself. You are unique and we are all ourselves. Everything happens for a reason. I have cancer for a reason; I think my research trial may help save other kids' lives.

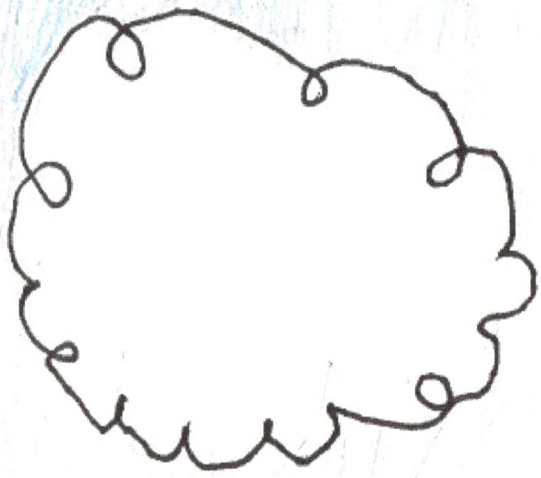

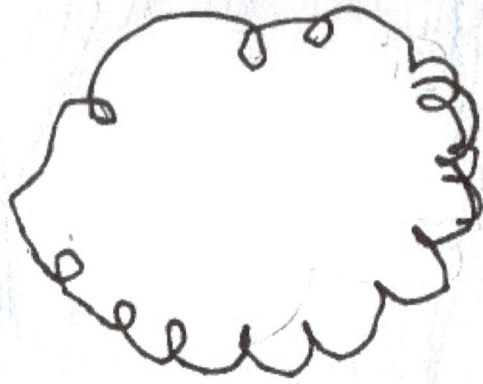

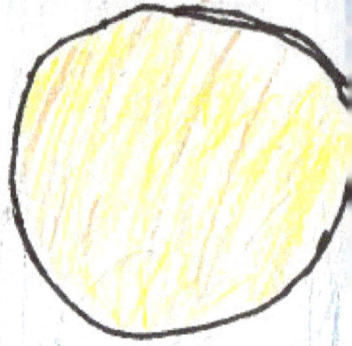

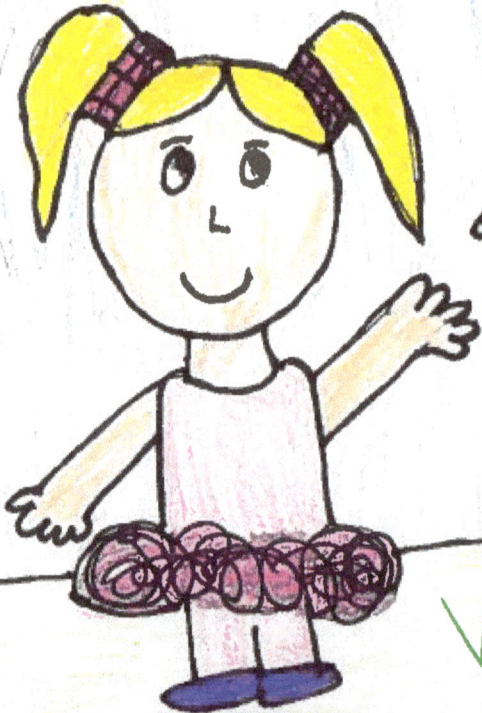

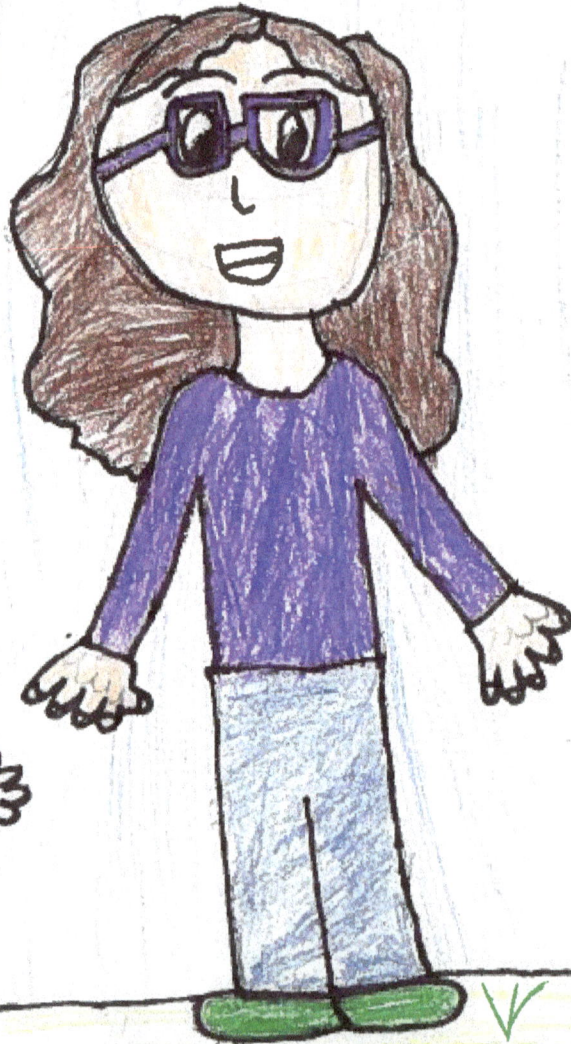

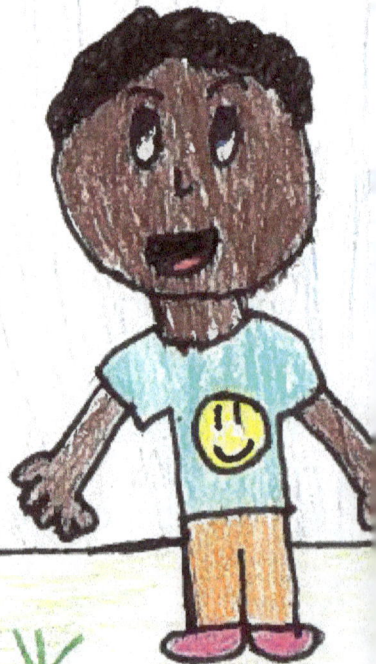

Vision changes in kindergarten

If something's wrong, tell a grown-up

Sometimes I wish I didn't have cancer

I believe in courage

On my golden 20th birthday,
   I want a huge party

No need for medicine someday

EMERSON'S STORY

My vision was a BIG concern in my cancer journey because it all started with some pressure on my eyes and double vision. That's when my mom took me to the hospital, and we found I have a rare, aggressive brain tumor.

My vision for the future is to be cancer free and to have my research help other kids be cancer free. When I grow up, I want to be a Child Life Specialist.

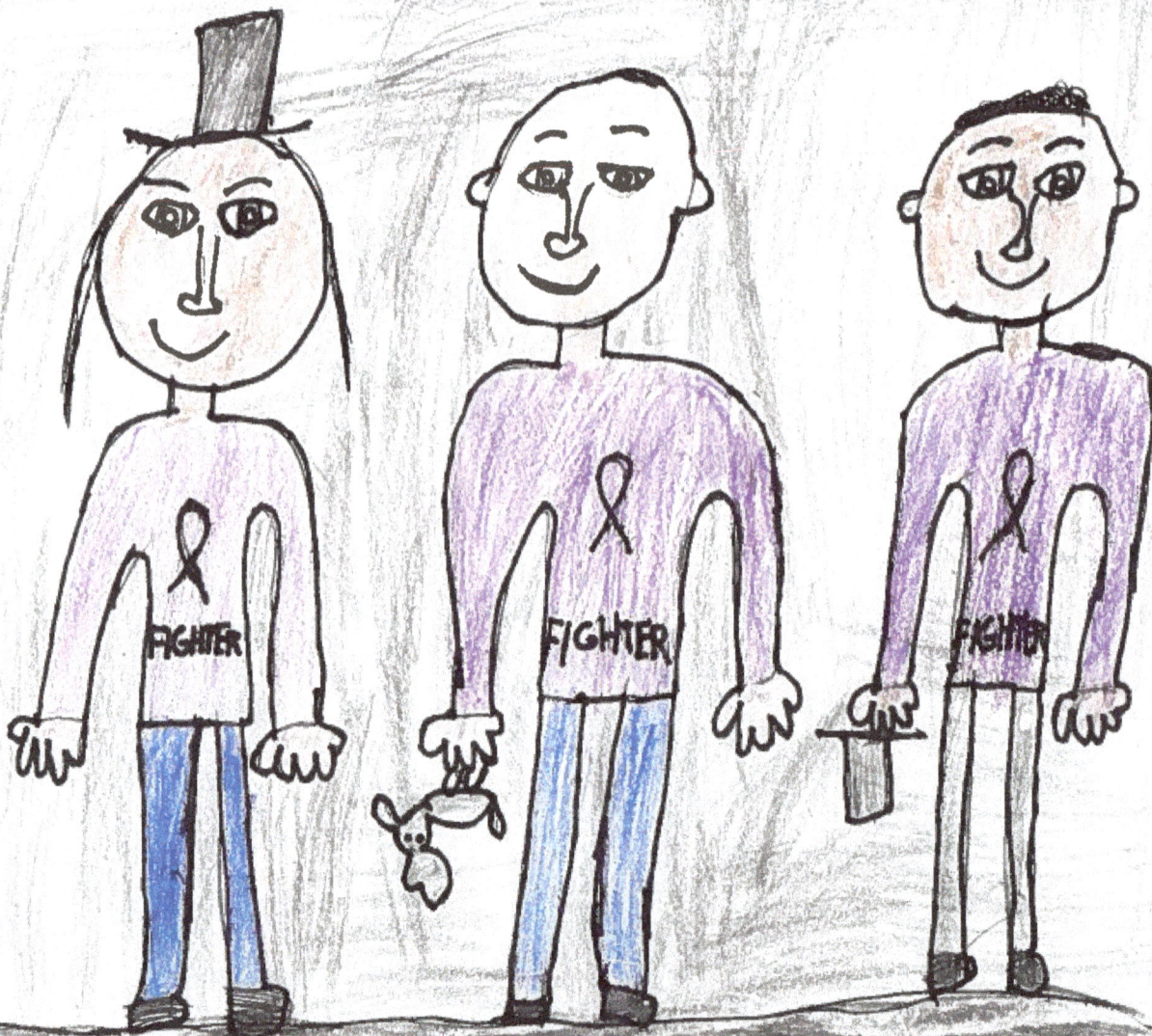

Will I be cancer free this year?

A warrior can face their fears
and has a lot of determination

Remember you aren't dying from
cancer, you are living with it

Rainbows always come after a storm

I am ready to be awesome

Overcoming fears was a huge part
of my journey

Really, you can do anything
you put your mind to

EMERSON'S STORY

It's not always easy to be a warrior. I cry all the time because of my cancer, which is embarrassing. Then I get up in the morning and keep going. I explain to my mom how I feel, and she says, "You got this." Even warriors need to cry and have feelings and lean on people.

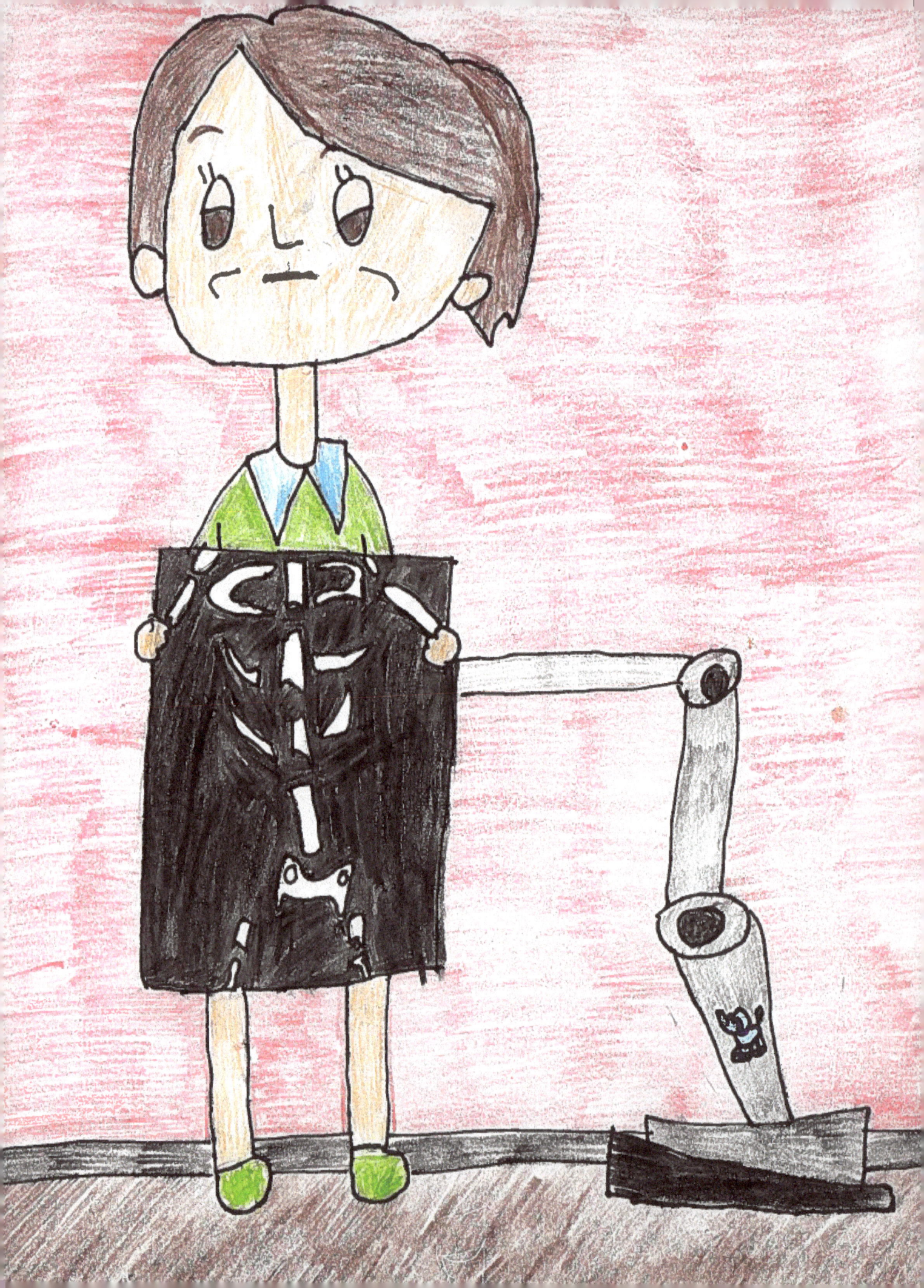

X

X-RAY

e**X**cited to see the pictures

Really hard to hold my breath

A look inside at my lungs

You wear a heavy vest so they only
x-ray the parts they need

EMERSON'S STORY

It feels like I've had billions of x-rays, too many to count! But they don't hurt. Just hold still and it's over quickly. The x-rays can show the doctors what is wrong and also when you're getting better.

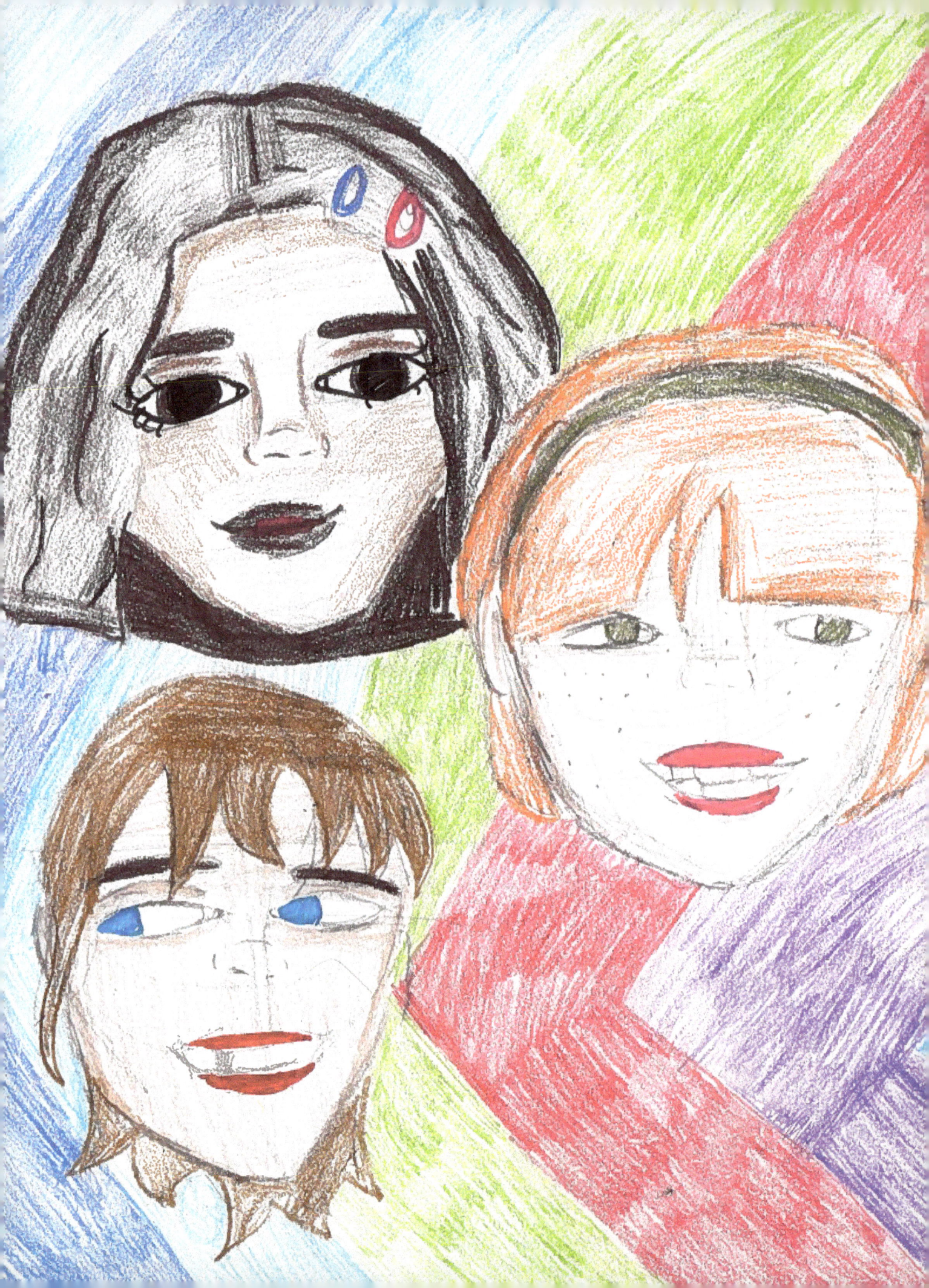

You can do this!

Overcoming your fears

U are unique in your own way; it's what's on the inside that counts

EMERSON'S STORY

Other kids might think they want to have cancer because they want attention. I'd rather have attention for things like being me, playing basketball and getting a basket, or being in a play and taking a bow. I want to be known because I'm kind and have good friends, not just as the girl who has cancer. I'm not my trial drug. I may have cancer, but that's not who I am. Remember, it's what YOU do and who YOU are that's important.

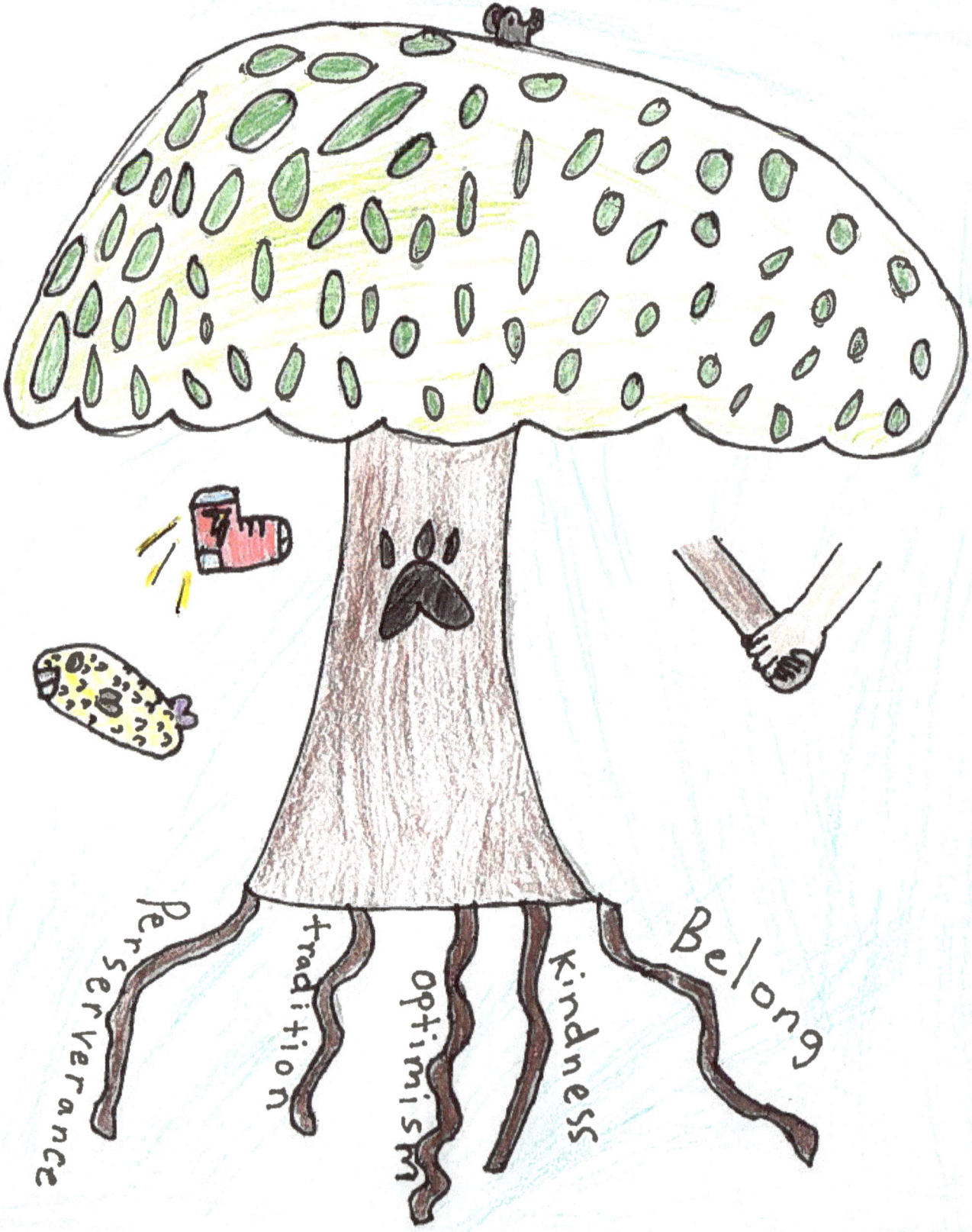

We are family!

All the teachers supporting me

Uniting together to help families

Kids willing to help

A lot of gifts and well-wishes from my friends

Zoo graduates playing for Purple Power games

Once in a while I would miss homework

Our chosen family

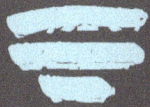

Z

EMERSON'S STORY

Waukazoo is my elementary school in Holland, Michigan. From the start to the finish of the first part of my cancer journey, they were there. Teachers came to our house to clean the leaves from our lawn, mow the grass, and do yard work, just to help when I was in the hospital. Friends from school have come to my cancer charity auction ever since it started. Some friends I've known since kindergarten and we're still friends. I hope your school can support you the way mine supported me!

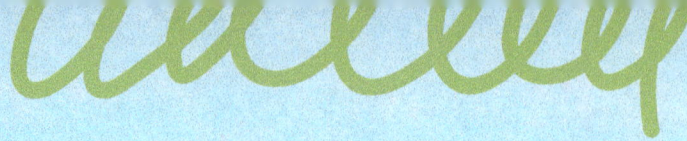

AFTERWORD

When I started this book, it was just a 4th grade school project. My cancer had been stable for five years. Then at the end of my 5th grade year, I found out that I had another brain tumor. But it's a totally different tumor. Dr. Koschmann described it like a bus stop where one kid got off (my first tumor) and another kid got on (my second tumor). Since I started middle school, I've had two new surgeries and started new treatments. My first tumor is still stable. And we're still treating the new ones.

In 6th grade, I love having multiple teachers and walking around the school. You get to spend time with other people at lunch, not just in your class. I love my new teachers, just like I loved my elementary school teachers.

With my grandma, it's kind of fun to go, just us together, to get my infusions. We like to craft too and use the Cricut. I like to help my mom with her classroom work. My little brother and I play Roblox and Minecraft. My little sister is one of my favorite people. We play baby dolls and Barbie dolls. She's teaching me how to care for the baby doll. I like to read to her.

I'm looking forward to not having to miss school, joining the knitting club with my cousin, being on the basketball team, learning to drive (I drive my grandma's golf cart!), vacations with my family, and going to college at U of M to become a Child Life Specialist. If I could travel anywhere else in the world, Canada (I've always wanted to see Canada since my grandpa would bring back cool things), Israel, and Mexico. My biggest wish or dream would be to help people by being a Child Life Specialist like they have helped me.

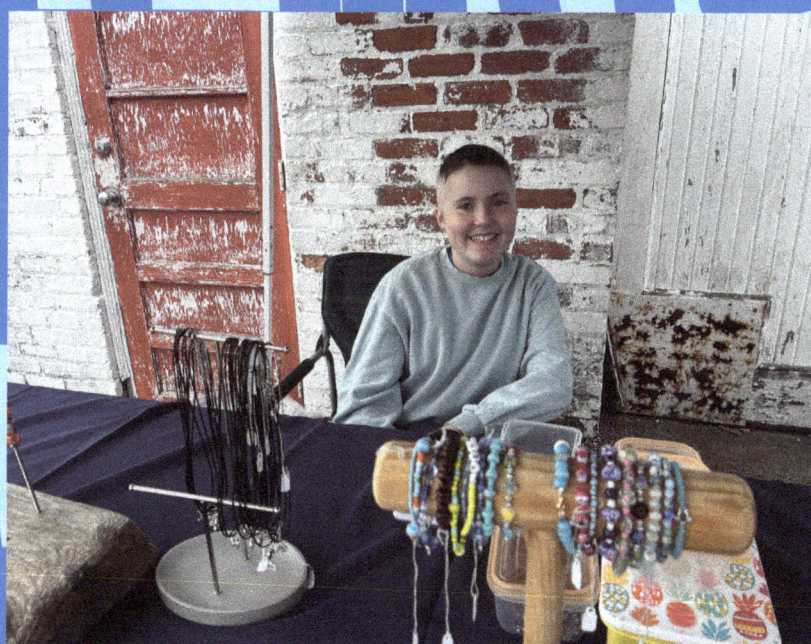

Emerson (6th grade) working at her charity event, Emerson-the-Brave, in September 2023

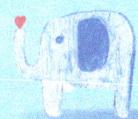

GLOSSARY

A — Ambulance

B — Bed

C — Child Life

D — Dr. Koschmann

E — Emergency

F — Food

G — Gifts

H — Helen DeVos

I — ICU

J — Journey

K — Knowledge

L — Laboratory

M — MRI

N — Nurses

O — Operation

P — Patient

Q — Question

R — Radiation

S — Surgery

T — Today

U — Unique

V — Visitors

W — Warrior

X — X-ray

Y — You

Z — WaukaZoo

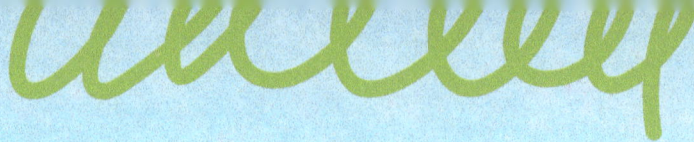

ACKNOWLEDGMENTS

I have many people to thank for helping me to write this book. First, thank you to my 4th grade teacher, Ms. Kovacs, for taking a student's dream and making it a reality! Thank you to Michael Kesterke, Carolyn Stich, and Anna McCuaig who became our book mentors and guided us through the process. Next, thank you to all my family and friends and teachers who read my drafts and asked for more of my personal story. Thank you to my cousin Avery Francis and my friends Elena de Alvare, Christian Bradley, Kora Hoisington, and Urijah Taylor for helping to illustrate my book. Also, thank you to Sarah Meiers and Mission Point Press for publishing my book and making it real. A huge thank you to all the doctors, nurses, Child Life Specialists, and medical staff at the University of Michigan and Helen DeVos hospitals who have cared for me since kindergarten, especially Dr. Carl Koschmann. I wouldn't be here without you. And finally, thank you to my parents and my grandparents who have always been there for me…no matter what. And to all the kids out there who also have cancer — I hope you have as many people who love and support you as I do!

"I was hoping to make this more about the reader than myself. You are unique and we are all ourselves. Everything happens for a reason. I have cancer for a reason: I think my research trial may help save other kids' lives."

— EMERSON

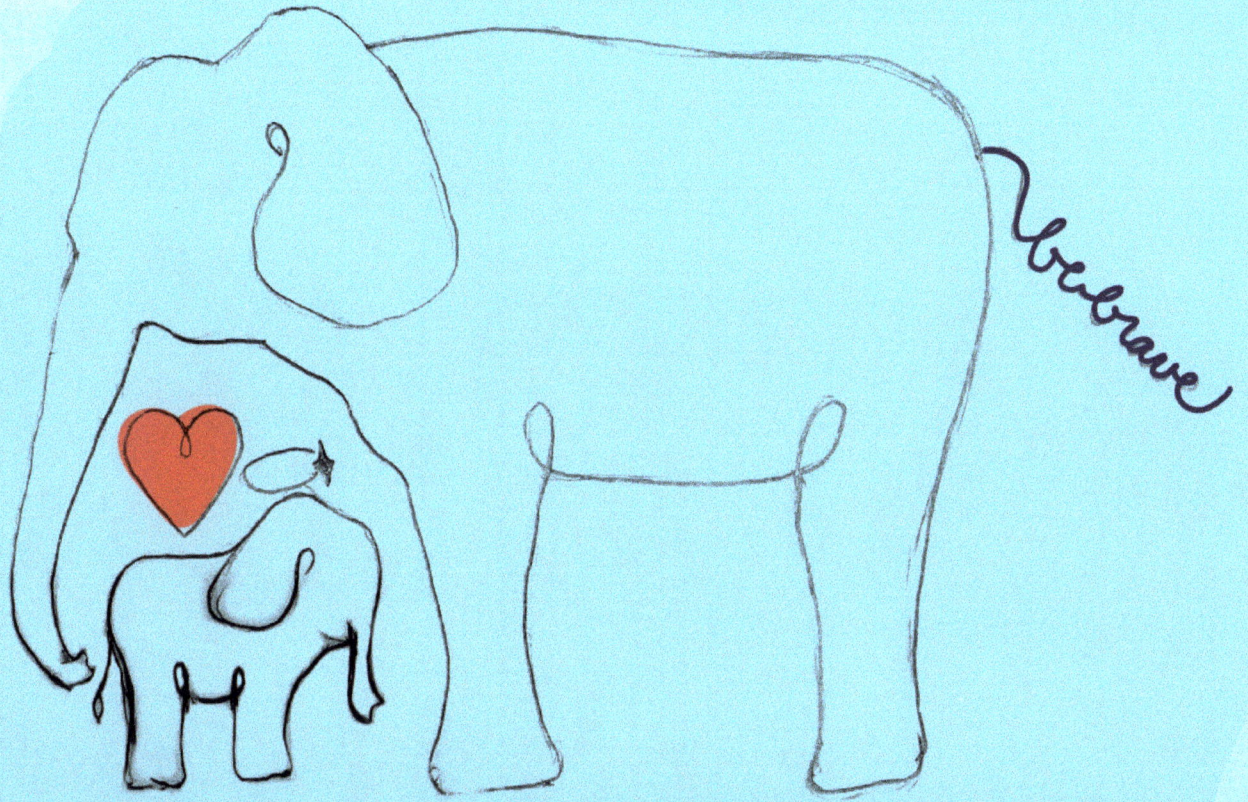

www.ingramcontent.com/pod-product-compliance
Lightning Source LLC
Chambersburg PA
CBHW052350210326
41597CB00038B/6321